KIDNEY STONE DIET COOKBOOK FOR SENIORS

Comprehensive Nutrition Strategies and Wholesome Recipes for Prevention, Management, and Lifelong Health

Dr. Kelly Haaland

Copyright © 2024 All rights reserved.

No part of this book may be reproduced or transmitted in any form or by any means, electronic or mechanical, including photocopying, recording, or by any information storage and retrieval system, without written permission from the author. The scanning, uploading, and distribution of this book via the internet or via any other means without the permission of the author is illegal and punishable by law. The author has made every effort to ensure the accuracy of the information contained in this book. However, the author cannot be held responsible for any errors or omissions.

Table of Contents

Introduction..7

Chapter 1: Kidney Stone Basics
What Are Kidney Stones?..9
Types of Kidney Stones..11
Causes and Risk Factors..13
Symptoms and When to Seek Help..15

Chapter 2: Dietary Management of Kidney Stones
The Role of Diet in Preventing Kidney Stones....................17
Foods to Eat and Avoid..20
Nutritional Considerations for Seniors..23

Breakfast Recipes
Low-Oxalate Berry Smoothie..26
Egg White Omelette..27
Oatmeal..28
Whole Wheat Toast..29
Banana Pancakes..30
Greek Yogurt Parfait..31
Cottage Cheese Bowl..32
Quinoa Porridge..33
Vegetable Stir-Fry..34
Rice Cakes..35
Buckwheat Pancakes..36
Muesli..37
Melon Salad..38
Zucchini Bread..39
Scrambled Tofu..40
Rice Pudding..41
Polenta..42

Shakshuka...43
Sweet Potato Hash..44
Veggie Breakfast Tacos..45
Pear and Walnut Oatmeal...46
Apple Cinnamon Quinoa Bowl.................................47
Pumpkin Seed Granola...48
Cornmeal Porridge..49
Almond Flour Biscuits..50
Berry and Flaxseed Smoothie..................................51

Lunch Recipes
Grilled Chicken Salad:..52
Lentil Soup..53
Quinoa Stuffed Bell Peppers....................................54
Turkey Wrap...55
Vegetarian Chili...56
Salmon and Arugula Salad.......................................57
Roasted Vegetable Plate..58
Pasta Primavera...59
Tofu Stir-Fry...60
Vegetable Curry...61
Egg Salad...62
Shrimp and Avocado Salad......................................63
Beet and Goat Cheese Salad...................................64
Rice and Bean Bowl...65
Tuna Salad...66
Caprese Salad..67
Grilled Veggie Sandwich..68
Soba Noodle Salad..69
Cauliflower Rice Stir-Fry..70
Kale and Quinoa Salad..71
Zucchini Noodle Bowl..72
Mushroom Risotto...73
Spinach and Feta Stuffed Salmon...........................74
Greek Lentil Salad...75
Chickpea Vegetable Patties....................................76

Vegetables

Roasted Cauliflower Steaks..77
Asparagus and Lemon Risotto..78
Brussels Sprouts with Balsamic Glaze..79
Stuffed Acorn Squash..80
Green Beans Almondine..81
Cucumber Tomato Salad..82
Balsamic Roasted Carrots..83
Zucchini Boats..84
Spinach and Mushroom Frittata...85
Kale Caesar Salad...86
Vegetable Paella..87
Mushroom Stroganoff..88
Broccoli and Almond Soup...89
Roasted Beet and Walnut Salad..90
Ratatouille...91
Leek and Potato Soup..92
Grilled Vegetable Platter..93
Sweet Potato Rounds...94
Collard Greens with Garlic...95
Artichoke and Spinach Dip...96
Roasted Parsnips with Rosemary...97

Desserts

Baked Apples..98
Pineapple Sorbet..99
Rice Pudding..100
Poached Pears..101
Angel Food Cake..102
Pumpkin Mousse...103
Lemon Jelly..104
Banana Ice Cream..105
Mango Pudding...106
Berry Salad...107
Apple Crisp..108
Almond Macaroons...109
Melon Balls..110

6-WEEK MEAL PLAN..111

To show our appreciation for your purchase, we're delighted to offer you these special bonuses as a heartfelt thank you.

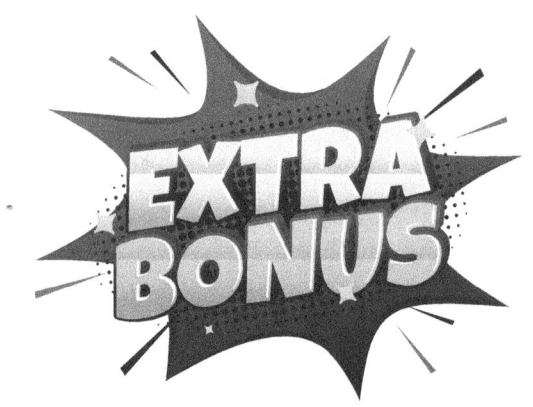 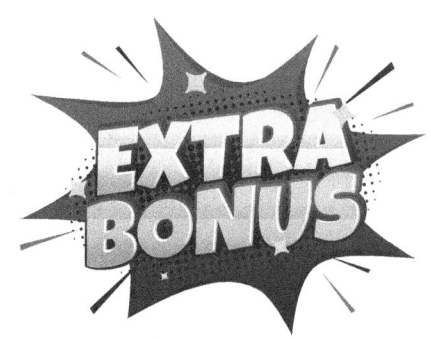

1. A Food Tracker Journal
2. Downloadable E-BOOK featuring full-color images of finished recipes
3. One-on-one consultation session with Dr. Kelly Haaland

Dear Esteemed Reader,

We recognize that each individual is as unique as the ingredients that make up a perfect dish. With this in mind, we gently remind you that the recipes within these pages are starting points on your path to a kidney stone-conscious diet. Your body's requirements are distinct, shaped by your health history, current condition, and the specific advice of your healthcare professionals. As such, we encourage you to use this cookbook as a flexible guide. Feel free to adjust the recipes to align with your personal dietary needs and preferences. Should a certain ingredient raise a question, or if a substitution is in order, we invite you to embrace the opportunity to tailor these dishes to suit your taste and health requirements perfectly.

Moreover, we acknowledge that nutrition is a science as much as it is an art. The nutritional information provided alongside each recipe is an approximate estimation, designed to assist you in making informed choices. Variations in ingredient types, brands, and the very act of culinary creation may lead to slight deviations in these nutritional figures. We encourage you to consider these numbers as helpful guides rather than strict mandates, allowing the joy of cooking to remain at the heart of your dietary journey. In moments of uncertainty or if a particular dietary concern arises, we strongly advocate for consulting with your doctor or a dietary specialist. These professionals can offer personalized advice, ensuring that your diet remains aligned with your health goals and medical needs. They are your partners in health, equipped to navigate the complexities of dietary management with you, especially when adjustments are needed.

Furthermore, If our cookbook has brought joy to your kitchen and table, we'd be thrilled to hear about your experiences in an Amazon review. On the flip side, if you stumble upon any hiccups while exploring our recipes, don't hesitate to get in touch at **kellyhaaland2@gmail.com** We're here to support your cooking journey every step of the way.

With warmest regards and best wishes for your health,
Dr. Kelly Haaland

Introduction

Welcome to the "Kidney Stone Diet Cookbook for Seniors" – your new companion in the kitchen and a trusted guide on your journey to better kidney health! If you or someone you love is navigating the challenges of kidney stones, particularly in the golden years, this book is a ray of sunshine. , offering not just recipes, but a new perspective on food and wellness.

Why a specialized cookbook for seniors, you might wonder? As we age, our bodies undergo various changes, and our dietary needs evolve. The risk of kidney stones increases, and managing this risk becomes crucial for maintaining a vibrant and active lifestyle. This book acknowledges the unique dietary considerations for seniors, blending them with preventive strategies against kidney stones. It's not just about what you can or cannot eat; it's about enjoying nutritious, delicious food that nurtures your body and soul. Kidney stones can be a daunting foe. They don't discriminate, affecting the young and the old, but seniors face distinct challenges. The pain, the discomfort, and the interruption to daily life – it's a lot to handle. But here's the good news: your diet is a powerful tool in your arsenal against kidney stones, and we're here to show you how to use it effectively. Our recipes are crafted to reduce the risk of stone formation, focusing on ingredients that support kidney health and overall well-being. But this book is more than just a collection of recipes. It's a manifesto for a healthier, happier life in your senior years. We delve into the science of kidney stones, breaking it down into understandable and actionable advice. You'll learn about the types of kidney stones, the role of hydration, and the importance of dietary balance. We demystify the oxalates, the calcium, the sodium, and the protein, guiding you on how to make informed choices about what you eat.

The recipes you'll discover here are thoughtfully designed with seniors in mind, considering not just kidney health but also common age-related conditions. They are easy to prepare, nutritionally balanced, and, most importantly, delicious. From hearty breakfasts to refreshing beverages, from comforting soups to scrumptious main courses, every recipe is a step towards a healthier you, minimizing the risk of kidney stones without sacrificing taste or enjoyment. Eating well should be a joy, not a chore. That's why we've prioritized variety, flavor, and simplicity. Whether you're cooking for one, two, or a whole family, you'll find dishes that satisfy your taste buds, nourish your body, and bring a smile to your face. Picture yourself starting the day with a smooth, creamy oatmeal, infused with antioxidant-rich berries, or sitting down to a dinner of tender grilled fish, seasoned to perfection and paired with a side of aromatic, kidney-friendly herbs. But what truly sets this cookbook apart is its commitment to empowering seniors with knowledge and skills. It's about transforming your relationship with food, embracing a diet that's not only preventive but also pleasurable. It's about making every meal a celebration of life, a testament to your commitment to your health and your enjoyment of the finer, flavorsome things in life.

So, whether you're a senior, a caregiver, or simply someone looking to support kidney health through diet, this cookbook is for you. It's time to turn the page, to start cooking, and to embark on a flavorful journey to better health. Welcome to the **"Kidney Stone Diet Cookbook for Seniors"** – where delicious food meets healthy living, crafted especially with you in mind.

Chapter 1: Kidney Stone Basics

What Are Kidney Stones?.

Kidney stones are hard deposits made of minerals and salts that form inside your kidneys. They can affect any part of your urinary tract — from your kidneys to your bladder — and are often painful when passing through the urinary system.

Understanding Kidney Stones

These stones form when the urine becomes concentrated, allowing minerals to crystallize and stick together. They can range in size from as small as a grain of sand to as large as a golf ball. Small stones might pass through the urinary tract without causing too much pain, but larger stones can block the flow of urine and cause severe pain or bleeding.

Composition of Kidney Stones

Kidney stones can be made up of various substances. The most common types include:
- Calcium stones
- Struvite stones
- Uric acid stones
- Cystine stones

Brief History

The problem of kidney stones has been recognized for millennia, with descriptions of surgical treatments dating back to ancient civilizations. Historical texts from Egypt, Greece, and Rome describe kidney stones, indicating their prevalence in ancient societies. In the past, treatments were primitive and often consisted of painful methods to remove stones. The famous Hippocratic Oath, originating from ancient Greece, even includes a passage where physicians swear not to perform surgery for stones, leaving the task to specialists of the time known as lithotomists.

The understanding and treatment of kidney stones have evolved significantly over centuries. The 20th century brought groundbreaking advancements, including the development of the lithotripter in the 1980s, a machine that uses shock waves to break up stones into small pieces that can be passed naturally. Today, the management of kidney stones includes a combination of lifestyle changes, medication, and various procedures that range from minimally invasive techniques to surgical removal, depending on the stone's size, composition, and location.

Types of Kidney Stones

There are four primary types of kidney stones, each with different causes and characteristics:

1. Calcium Stones

- **Calcium oxalate:** The most common type of kidney stone, which forms when calcium combines with oxalate in the urine. Insufficient fluid intake, a high-protein diet, and certain genetic predispositions can increase the concentration of calcium or oxalate in urine, leading to the formation of these stones. Factors like high doses of vitamin D, intestinal bypass surgery, and several metabolic disorders can also increase the concentration of calcium or oxalate in urine.
- **Calcium phosphate:** Less common than calcium oxalate stones, these form in alkaline urine. They can be associated with certain metabolic conditions, such as renal tubular acidosis, and can sometimes occur in those who take medications to treat migraines or seizures.

2. Uric Acid Stones

These stones form when the urine is consistently acidic. Diets high in purines—substances found in animal protein such as meats, fish, and shellfish—can increase uric acid in urine. When uric acid becomes concentrated in urine, it can settle and form a stone by itself or along with calcium. People with gout or those undergoing chemotherapy are at higher risk for developing uric acid stones.

3. Struvite Stones

Struvite stones are typically associated with urinary tract infections. They can grow quickly and become quite large, sometimes with few symptoms or little warning. These stones are a mix of magnesium, ammonium, and phosphate, and their formation can be linked to an infection by bacteria that produce urease, an enzyme that increases the urine pH and leads to stone formation.

4. Cystine Stones

These are rare and form in individuals with a hereditary disorder called cystinuria, which affects the kidneys' ability to reabsorb certain amino acids from the urine. As a result, excessive amounts of cystine accumulate in the urine, leading to the formation of cystine stones. These stones can be larger and are often difficult to treat.

Treatment and Prevention

The treatment for kidney stones varies depending on the stone type:

- **Calcium stones:** Often treated with medication to decrease the production of calcium or oxalate in the urine and recommendations for dietary changes, such as reducing sodium and animal protein.
- **Uric acid stones:** Treated with medications that alkalize the urine, dietary adjustments to reduce purine intake, and measures to increase fluid intake.
- **Struvite stones:** Management often involves treating the underlying urinary tract infections and may require surgical removal of the stone.
- **Cystine stones:** Treatment includes a high fluid intake, medications to reduce cystine concentration in the urine, and sometimes dietary adjustments.

Preventive strategies are tailored to the stone type but generally include staying well-hydrated, making dietary changes, and, in some cases, taking medications to correct the conditions that contribute to stone formation.

Causes and Risk Factors

Causes of Kidney Stones

The formation of kidney stones occurs when there are more crystal-forming substances in the urine, such as calcium, oxalate, and uric acid, than the fluid in your urine can dilute. At the same time, your urine may lack substances that prevent crystals from sticking together, creating an ideal environment for kidney stones to form. These conditions can result from various factors, including:

- **Dehydration:** Not drinking enough water each day can increase your risk of kidney stones. People in warm climates and those who sweat a lot may be at higher risk.
- **Diet:** A diet high in protein, sodium (salt), and sugar can increase the chance of some types of kidney stones. This is especially true with a high-sodium diet, which can increase the amount of calcium your kidneys must filter, thus increasing the risk of kidney stones.
- **Digestive diseases and surgery:** Gastric bypass surgery, inflammatory bowel disease, or chronic diarrhea can cause changes in the digestive process that affect your absorption of calcium and water, increasing the levels of stone-forming substances in your urine.

Risk Factors

Several factors can increase your risk of developing kidney stones:

- **Family or personal history:** If someone in your family has had kidney stones, you're more likely to develop stones, too. If you've already had one or more kidney stones, you're at increased risk of developing another.
- **Dehydration:** Not drinking enough fluids, especially water, is a common contributor to kidney stone formation.

- **Certain diets:** Eating a diet that's high in protein, sodium, and sugar may increase the risk of some types of kidney stones. This is particularly true for high sodium intake, which can increase calcium kidney stone risk.
- **Obesity:** High body mass index (BMI), large waist size, and weight gain have been linked to an increased risk of kidney stones.
- **Medical conditions:** Conditions such as renal tubular acidosis, cystinuria, hyperparathyroidism, certain urinary tract infections, and other medical conditions can increase the risk of kidney stones.
- **Supplements and medications:** Using vitamin C supplements, dietary supplements, and certain medications like diuretics (water pills), anti-seizure drugs, and calcium-based antacids may increase the risk of stones.
- **Other factors:** Factors like being of a certain age (20s-50s), gender (more common in men than women), and a sedentary lifestyle can also contribute to the risk of kidney stone formation.

Symptoms and When to Seek Help..

Kidney stones are notorious for being painful, but they can also present with various other symptoms. Understanding these can help in recognizing when it's time to seek medical assistance.

Symptoms of Kidney Stones
The symptoms of kidney stones can vary, often depending on the size of the stone, its location, and whether it obstructs the urinary tract. Common symptoms include:
- **Severe pain:** The most characteristic symptom is intense pain, known as renal colic. This pain can start suddenly and might fluctuate in intensity. It's typically felt in the side and back, below the ribs, and can radiate to the lower abdomen and groin. The nature of the pain can be sharp, stabbing, and comes in waves.
- **Pain during urination:** This is often experienced when the stone is passing through the ureter and nearing the bladder, causing irritation and a burning sensation similar to a urinary tract infection.
- **Cloudy or foul-smelling urine:** The presence of a stone can cause urine to become cloudy or have a strong, unpleasant odor due to infection.
- **Blood in the urine (hematuria):** This can be visible (red, pink, or brown urine) or microscopic and is a common symptom, resulting from the stone irritating the kidneys or other parts of the urinary tract.
- **Frequent urination or urge to urinate:** Changes in frequency or urgency can occur when a stone is lodged in the ureter, creating an irritation that mimics the need to urinate more often.

- **Nausea and vomiting:** These symptoms can occur due to the intense pain of the kidney stones and are often a body's response to significant discomfort.
- **Fever and chills:** If an infection is present in the urinary tract along with the stone, fever and chills might develop, indicating a more serious condition that requires immediate attention.

Timely medical evaluation is essential for anyone exhibiting these symptoms, as kidney stones can lead to significant complications if not treated properly. Depending on the situation, treatment might involve pain relief, medication to help the stone pass, or various procedures to remove or break up the stone. If you're experiencing any of the above symptoms or suspect you have kidney stones, consult with a healthcare provider for an accurate diagnosis and appropriate management.

Chapter 2: Dietary Management of Kidney Stones

The Role of Diet in Preventing Kidney Stones.

Diet plays a pivotal role in the prevention of kidney stones, significantly influencing their likelihood of forming. A well-planned diet can reduce the risk of certain types of stones, considering that the composition and quantity of substances like calcium, oxalate, uric acid, and phosphate in the urine are heavily affected by dietary choices.

Understanding the Connection
Kidney stones form when certain substances in urine, like calcium, oxalate, uric acid, and phosphate, become highly concentrated. Diet affects this concentration by influencing the balance of these substances and the overall chemical environment in the urinary system.

Key Dietary Strategies
1. Stay Hydrated
- Water Intake: Drinking plenty of fluids, especially water, is one of the most effective measures to prevent kidney stones. Fluids dilute the substances in urine that lead to stones. Aim for at least 2 to 3 liters of fluid daily, more if you live in a hot climate or lead an active lifestyle.

2. Calcium Intake
- Balanced Consumption: While it might seem counterintuitive, a diet low in calcium can actually increase the risk of developing calcium oxalate stones. Adequate dietary calcium helps decrease the amount of oxalate being absorbed by your body, so it's crucial to consume an appropriate amount, ideally through food sources like dairy products, leafy greens, and fortified foods.

3. **Reduce Oxalate-Rich Foods**
   - **Selective Reduction:** If you're prone to forming calcium oxalate stones, your doctor might recommend a diet low in oxalate. Foods rich in oxalate include spinach, beets, nuts, chocolate, tea, and certain fruits like strawberries and rhubarb.
4. **Limit Salt and Animal Protein**
   - **Sodium Reduction:** A high-salt diet can trigger kidney stones because it increases the amount of calcium in the urine. Opt for a low-sodium diet by reducing processed foods, fast foods, and salty snacks.
   - **Animal Protein Moderation:** Diets high in animal protein (meat, poultry, fish, and eggs) can increase the risk of kidney stones. High protein intake can reduce levels of citrate, the chemical in urine that helps prevent stones from forming, and increase uric acid, which could lead to stone formation.
5. **Control Uric Acid Levels**
   - **Limit Purines:** Foods high in purines, such as red meat, organ meats, and shellfish, can increase uric acid in urine. If you are prone to uric acid stones, consider reducing your intake of these foods.

Special Considerations
- **Potassium Intake:** A diet rich in potassium can help prevent the formation of kidney stones, particularly if you are prone to developing calcium oxalate stones. Foods like bananas, oranges, and sweet potatoes are high in potassium.
- **Alkaline Diet:** An alkaline diet, rich in fruits and vegetables and lower in meat and grains, can help reduce the risk of uric acid stones and may help prevent calcium stones.

Individualized Diet Plans

It's important to remember that dietary recommendations can vary based on the type of kidney stones you're prone to forming and your individual health profile. Consulting with a healthcare professional or a dietitian can provide personalized dietary advice, ensuring that you're taking the right steps to prevent kidney stones while maintaining overall health.

Foods to Eat and Avoid

Managing your diet is a key strategy in preventing kidney stones. Depending on the type of stones you are prone to, certain foods can either promote or reduce your risk. A thorough guide is provided here on what foods to eat and avoid to help manage the risk of kidney stone formation.

Foods to Eat

1. Calcium-Rich Foods
   - Opt for: Dairy products like milk, cheese, and yogurt; plant-based sources like broccoli, kale, and tofu; and fortified foods.
   - Why: Adequate calcium intake can bind with oxalates in the foods you eat, reducing the risk of calcium oxalate stones.
2. Fluids
   - Opt for: Water is best; lemonade and orange juice can also be beneficial.
   - Why: Fluids dilute the substances in urine that lead to stones. Citrate-rich fluids like lemonade and orange juice may help prevent stone formation by binding with calcium in the urine.
3. Fruits and Vegetables
   - Opt for: A variety of fruits and vegetables, especially those rich in citrate, like lemons, oranges, and melons.
   - Why: They increase urine volume and citrate, a stone inhibitor, and provide fiber, which may help to reduce the risk of stone formation.
4. Whole Grains
   - Opt for: Brown rice, quinoa, oats, and whole wheat bread and pasta.
   - Why: Whole grains offer magnesium, which can help prevent the formation of crystals in the urine.

Foods to Avoid or Limit

1. **Oxalate-Rich Foods (for calcium oxalate stones)**
   - **Limit:** Spinach, rhubarb, almonds, beets, potatoes, and chocolate.
   - **Why:** These foods are high in oxalates, which can contribute to the formation of calcium oxalate stones.

2. **High-Sodium Foods**
   - **Limit:** Processed foods, canned soups, and fast foods.
   - **Why:** High sodium intake can increase calcium in the urine, which contributes to the formation of kidney stones.

3. **Animal Proteins**
   - **Limit:** Red meat, poultry, pork, and seafood.
   - **Why:** Excessive intake can increase uric acid, reduce citrate excretion, and raise the risk of stone formation.

4. **High-Sugar Foods**
   - **Limit:** Sodas, sweetened beverages, and candies.
   - **Why:** Sugar can increase kidney stone risk, possibly by increasing the size of the kidneys and changing the composition of the urine.

5. **Alcohol**
   - **Limit:** Especially beer and grain alcohols.
   - **Why:** Alcohol can lead to dehydration, concentrating the minerals in the urine and potentially leading to stone formation.

Additional Tips

- **Balance Oxalate Intake:** If you're prone to calcium oxalate stones, it's not necessary to completely avoid all oxalate-rich foods, but rather to consume them in moderation and pair them with calcium-rich foods to prevent oxalate absorption.
- **Limit Vitamin C Supplements:** Excessive vitamin C can convert to oxalate in the body, so be cautious with supplementation.

Monitor Salt and Sugar Substitutes: Some salt substitutes or "lite" salts are high in potassium, which can be problematic if you need to avoid oxalate or have other health issues. Also, some sugar substitutes can lead to diarrhea, which can contribute to stone formation if it results in dehydration.

It's important to tailor your diet based on the type of kidney stones you are prone to and your overall health. Consulting with a healthcare professional or a dietitian can provide personalized advice, ensuring that your diet supports your health while helping prevent the formation of kidney stones. An individualized approach is key, as dietary needs can vary widely based on personal health history, the type of stones, and other factors like medications and overall dietary patterns.

Nutritional Considerations for Seniors

Nutritional considerations for seniors with kidney stones are crucial since aging can influence the body's response to diet and its ability to process certain nutrients. Elderly individuals may have unique health challenges and dietary needs that require careful planning to prevent kidney stones while ensuring overall nutritional adequacy.

Hydration
- Importance: Adequate hydration is essential for preventing kidney stone formation, especially in seniors, who may have a diminished sense of thirst.
- Recommendation: Encourage regular fluid intake, aiming for at least 2 liters of water per day, unless contraindicated due to heart or kidney failure. Clear, pale urine is a good indicator of proper hydration.

Calcium Intake
- Importance: Seniors need adequate calcium to prevent osteoporosis, but balance is key, as too much can contribute to the risk of calcium stones.
- Recommendation: Obtain calcium from dietary sources like dairy products, green leafy vegetables, and fortified foods, rather than supplements, which have been linked to stone risk. The intake should be in line with recommended daily allowances, avoiding underconsumption or excessive intake.

Oxalate Management
- Importance: Limiting oxalate-rich foods can help reduce the risk of calcium oxalate stones, the most common type of kidney stones.
- Recommendation: Moderating high-oxalate foods like spinach, rhubarb, and almonds, especially if calcium oxalate stones are a concern. Combining oxalate-rich foods with calcium-rich foods can help reduce oxalate absorption.

Protein Moderation
- **Importance:** Excessive intake of animal protein can increase the risk of stone formation and can lead to decreased kidney function, a concern in the elderly.
- **Recommendation:** Opt for moderate portions of protein, prioritizing plant-based sources and lean meats, and avoiding high-protein diets.

Sodium Reduction
- **Importance:** High sodium intake can increase calcium excretion, contributing to the formation of kidney stones.
- **Recommendation:** Limit high-sodium foods like processed foods, canned soups, and salted snacks. Aim for a low-sodium diet as per dietary guidelines.

Potassium and Magnesium
- **Importance:** Both minerals can help reduce the risk of stone formation; potassium citrate is especially known for preventing certain types of stones.
- **Recommendation:** Include foods rich in potassium (like bananas, oranges, and potatoes) and magnesium (like nuts, seeds, and whole grains), unless contraindicated due to other medical conditions.

Uric Acid Stones Consideration
- **Importance:** Seniors with a history of uric acid stones should consider their purine intake.
- **Recommendation:** Limit purine-rich foods (such as red meat, organ meats, and shellfish) to reduce uric acid levels and the risk of uric acid stones.

Regular Dietary Reviews
- **Importance:** Nutritional needs and health status can change over time, especially in seniors.
- **Recommendation:** Regular consultations with healthcare providers or dietitians to adjust dietary plans as needed and to ensure that the diet is balanced and supports overall health without increasing the risk of stones.

Addressing Individual Needs
- **Consideration:** Each senior's health status, medication profile, and nutritional requirements are unique, especially concerning chronic conditions that can affect kidney stone risk, like diabetes and hypertension.
- **Action:** Personalize dietary plans based on individual health assessments, considering all medical conditions, medications, and the overall nutritional status.

Hence, nutritional management for seniors with kidney stones should focus on maintaining a balanced diet that supports overall health while preventing the formation of new stones. This includes staying hydrated, balancing calcium intake, moderating intake of oxalate and animal proteins, reducing sodium, and considering the individual's health needs. Regular check-ups with healthcare professionals are essential to tailor dietary recommendations and to monitor the overall health and kidney function of the elderly.

Breakfast Recipes

1. Low-Oxalate Berry Smoothie

Ingredients:
- 1 cup fresh blueberries (low in oxalates)
- 1 ripe banana
- 1 cup almond milk (calcium-fortified)
- 1 tablespoon honey (optional)
- ½ cup ice cubes

Instructions:
1. Combine the blueberries, banana, almond milk, and honey (if using) in a blender.
2. Add the ice cubes.
3. Blend on high until smooth and creamy.

Serves:
- 2 servings

Nutritional Info (per serving):
- Calories: 150
- Protein: 2g
- Carbohydrates: 36g
- Fat: 1.5g
- Fiber: 4g
- Calcium: 200mg

Cooking Time:
- Prep & Blend Time: 5 minutes

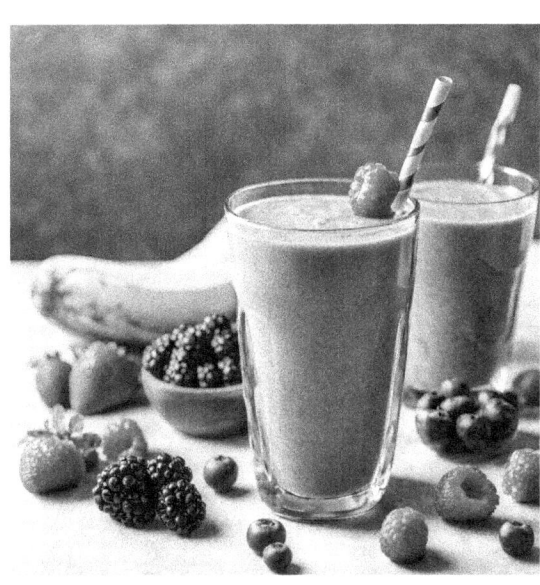

2. Egg White Omelette

Ingredients:
- 4 egg whites
- 1/2 cup chopped spinach (low oxalate)
- 1/4 cup diced bell peppers
- 2 tablespoons shredded low-fat cheese
- Salt and pepper to taste
- 1 teaspoon olive oil

Instructions:
1. Heat olive oil in a non-stick skillet over medium heat.
2. Whisk the egg whites in a bowl, and pour them into the skillet.
3. As the _____ a and tilt the pa_____
4. Sprinkl_____ alf of the omele_____
5. Fold t_____ minute.
6. Slide t_____

Serves:
- 1 servi_____

Nutrition_____
- Calori_____
- Protei_____
- Carbo_____
- Fat: 8g_____
- Fiber: _____
- Calciu_____

Cooking _____
- Prep & _____

27

3. Oatmeal

Ingredients:
- 1 cup rolled oats
- 2 cups water or low-fat milk
- Pinch of salt
- 1 tablespoon maple syrup or honey (optional)
- Fresh fruits (low-oxalate options like apples or bananas) for topping

Instructions:
1. Bring water or milk to a boil in a medium saucepan.
2. Add the oats and a pinch of salt, then reduce heat to low.
3. Simmer uncovered for 5 minutes, stirring occasionally.
4. Remove from heat and let stand for a couple of minutes.
5. Serve hot, topped with maple syrup or honey (if using) and fresh fruits.

Serves:
- 2 servings

Nutritional Info (per serving with water):
- Calories: 155
- Protein: 5g
- Carbohydrates: 27g
- Fat: 3g
- Fiber: 4g
- Calcium: 21mg

Cooking Time:
- Prep & Cook Time: 10 minutes

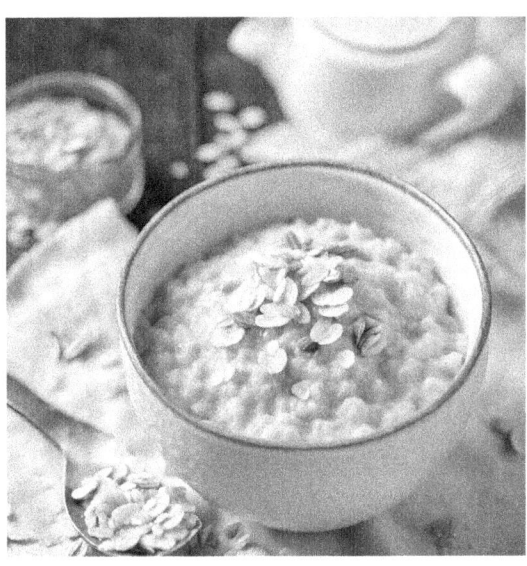

4. Whole Wheat Toast

Ingredients:
- 2 slices of whole wheat bread
- Your choice of low-oxalate toppings: almond butter, low-fat cream cheese, or avocado slices

Instructions:
1. Toast the whole wheat bread slices to your preferred level of crispiness.
2. Spread your chosen topping evenly over the toasted slices.

Serves:
- 1 serving

Nutritional Info (per serving with almond butter):
- Calories: 200
- Protein: 8g
- Carbohydrates: 18g
- Fat: 11g
- Fiber: 6g
- Calcium: 80mg

Cooking Time:
- Prep Time: 5 minutes

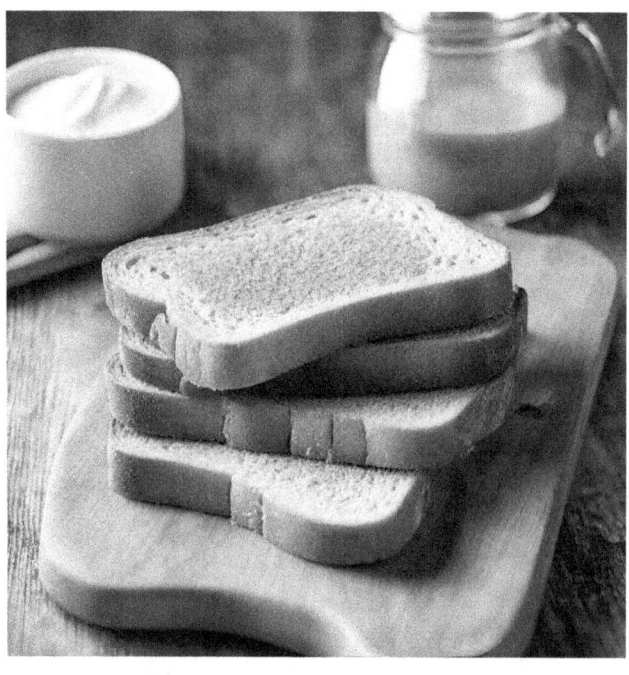

5. Banana Pancakes

Ingredients:
- 2 ripe bananas, mashed
- 2 eggs
- 1/2 cup whole wheat flour
- 1 tsp baking powder
- 1/2 tsp cinnamon
- 1/4 cup milk
- Butter or oil for cooking

Instructions:
1. In a bowl, combine the mashed bananas, eggs, and milk.
2. In another bowl, mix the whole wheat flour, baking powder, and cinnamon.
3. Fold the dry ingredients into the wet ingredients until just combined.
4. Heat a non-stick skillet over medium heat and brush with butter or oil.
5. Pour 1/4 cup of batter for each pancake and cook until bubbles form, then flip and cook until golden brown.

Serves:
- 2-3 servings

Nutritional Info (per serving):
- Calories: 280
- Protein: 9g
- Carbohydrates: 50g
- Fat: 6g
- Fiber: 6g
- Calcium: 60mg

Cooking Time:
- Prep & Cook Time: 20 minutes

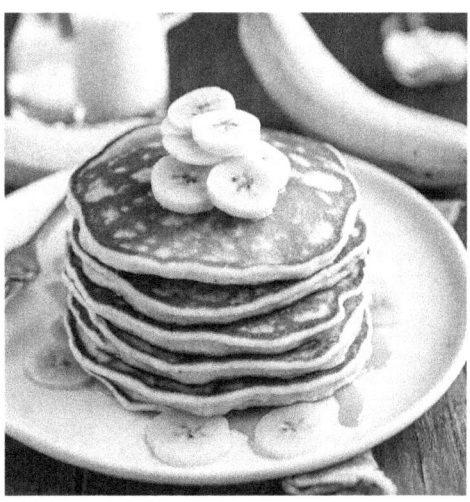

6. Greek Yogurt Parfait

Ingredients:
- 1 cup Greek yogurt (low-fat)
- 1/2 cup granola (low sugar, no added nuts or high-oxalate ingredients)
- 1 cup mixed berries (strawberries, blueberries, raspberries)
- 1 tbsp honey or maple syrup (optional)

Instructions:
1. In a glass or bowl, layer half the Greek yogurt.
2. Add a layer of half the granola and then half the berries.
3. Repeat the layers with the remaining ingredients.
4. Drizzle with honey or maple syrup if desired.

Serves:
- 1 serving

Nutritional Info (per serving):
- Calories: 350
- Protein: 25g
- Carbohydrates: 50g
- Fat: 7g
- Fiber: 5g
- Calcium: 200mg

Cooking Time:
- Prep Time: 10 minutes

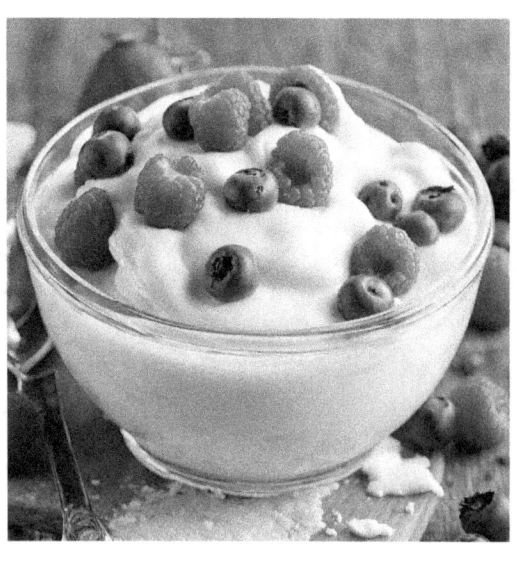

7. Cottage Cheese Bowl

Ingredients:
- 1 cup low-fat cottage cheese
- 1/2 cup pineapple chunks (fresh or canned in juice)
- 1/4 cup slivered almonds (optional, ensure low oxalate)
- 1 tablespoon honey or maple syrup

Instructions:
1. Place the cottage cheese in a serving bowl.
2. Top with pineapple chunks and slivered almonds if using.
3. Drizzle with honey or maple syrup.

Serves:
- 1 serving

Nutritional Info (per serving):
- Calories: 280
- Protein: 28g
- Carbohydrates: 35g
- Fat: 6g
- Fiber: 2g
- Calcium: 150mg

Cooking Time:
- Prep Time: 5 minutes

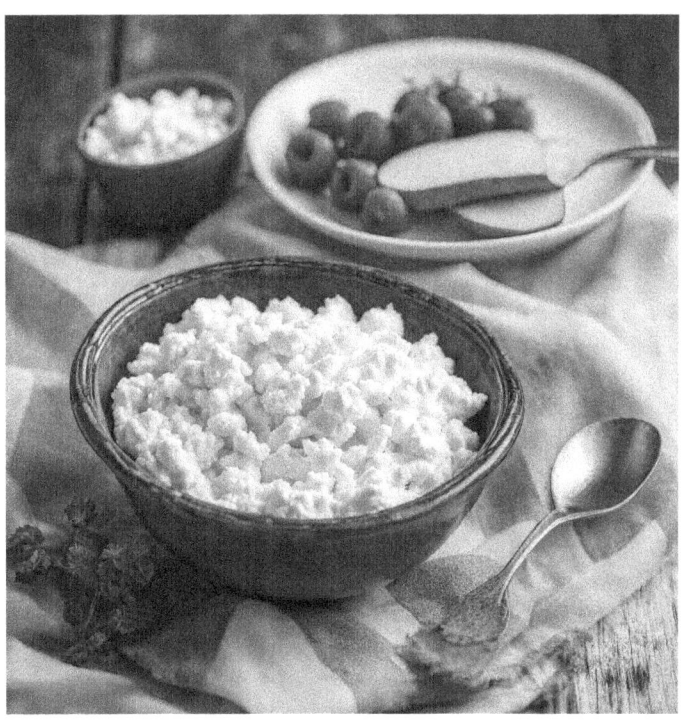

8. Quinoa Porridge

Ingredients:
- 1 cup quinoa, rinsed
- 2 cups almond milk
- 1 cinnamon stick or 1/2 tsp ground cinnamon
- 2 tbsp maple syrup or honey
- Fresh berries and sliced banana for topping

Instructions:
1. Combine quinoa, almond milk, and cinnamon in a saucepan and bring to a boil.
2. Reduce heat to low, cover, and simmer for 15 minutes or until most of the liquid is absorbed.
3. Remove from heat and let it sit covered for 5 minutes.
4. Stir in maple syrup or honey.
5. Serve hot topped with fresh berries and banana slices.

Serves:
- 2 servings

Nutritional Info (per serving):
- Calories: 320
- Protein: 8g
- Carbohydrates: 60g
- Fat: 5g
- Fiber: 5g
- Calcium: 150mg

Cooking Time:
- Prep & Cook Time: 25 minutes

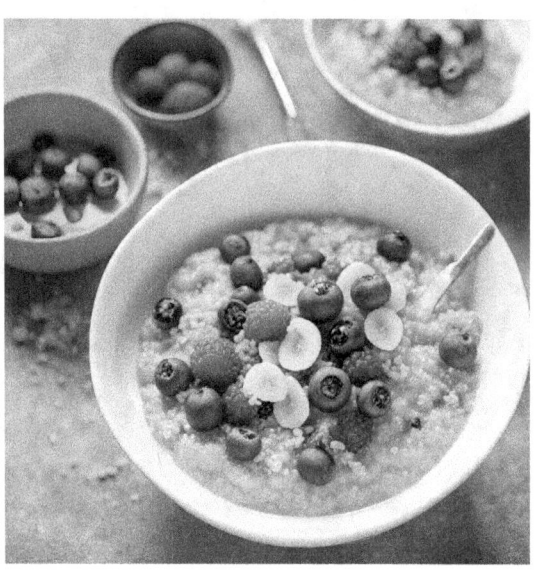

9. Vegetable Stir-Fry

Ingredients:
- 2 cups mixed vegetables (e.g., bell peppers, zucchini, carrots, broccoli - choose low-oxalate veggies)
- 1 tbsp olive oil
- 2 cloves garlic, minced
- 1 tbsp soy sauce (or tamari for gluten-free)
- 1 tsp ginger, grated
- 1/2 tsp black pepper
- 1/2 cup cooked brown rice or quinoa, to serve

Instructions:
1. Heat olive oil in a large skillet over medium-high heat.
2. Add garlic and ginger, sautéing for 30 seconds.
3. Add the mixed vegetables and stir-fry for 5-7 minutes until tender-crisp.
4. Stir in soy sauce (or tamari) and black pepper, cooking for an additional 1-2 minutes.
5. Serve the stir-fried vegetables hot over cooked brown rice or quinoa.

Serves:
- 2 servings

Nutritional Info (per serving):
- Calories: 250
- Protein: 6g
- Carbohydrates: 35g
- Fat: 10g
- Fiber: 8g
- Calcium: 40mg

Cooking Time:
- Prep & Cook Time: 20 minutes

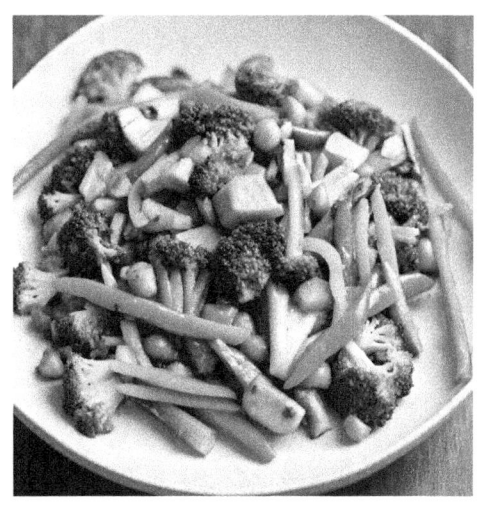

10. Rice Cakes

Ingredients:
- 4 plain rice cakes
- 2 tablespoons almond butter (or any low-oxalate nut butter)
- 1 banana, sliced
- 1 tablespoon chia seeds (optional)

Instructions:
1. Spread almond butter evenly over the rice cakes.
2. Top each rice cake with sliced banana.
3. Sprinkle chia seeds over the top, if using.

Serves:
- 2 servings (2 rice cakes per serving)

Nutritional Info (per serving):
- Calories: 300
- Protein: 8g
- Carbohydrates: 45g
- Fat: 10g
- Fiber: 7g
- Calcium: 50mg

Cooking Time:
- Prep Time: 5 minutes

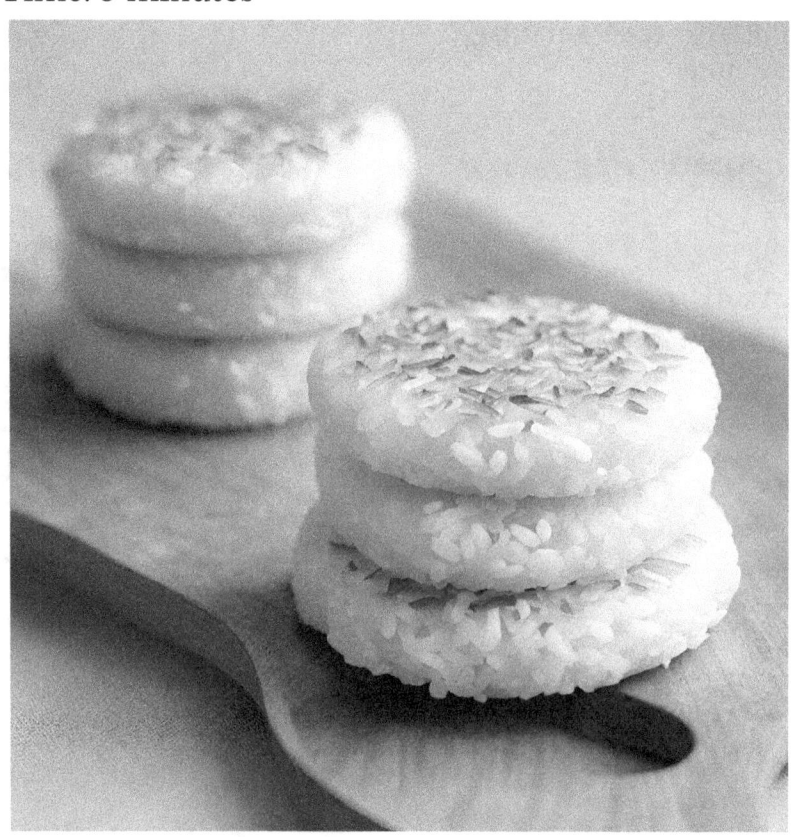

11. Buckwheat Pancakes

Ingredients:
- 1 cup buckwheat flour
- 1 tablespoon sugar (optional)
- 1 teaspoon baking powder
- 1/2 teaspoon salt
- 1 egg, beaten
- 1 cup milk
- 2 tablespoons melted butter or oil

Instructions:
1. In a large bowl, mix together the buckwheat flour, sugar, baking powder, and salt.
2. In another bowl, combine the beaten egg, milk, and melted butter.
3. Pour the wet ingredients into the dry ingredients and stir until just combined.
4. Heat a lightly oiled griddle or frying pan over medium-high heat.
5. Pour or scoop the batter onto the griddle, using approximately 1/4 cup for each pancake. Brown on both sides.

Serves:
- 3-4 servings

Nutritional Info (per serving):
- Calories: 220
- Protein: 8g
- Carbohydrates: 32g
- Fat: 7g
- Fiber: 5g
- Calcium: 90mg

Cooking Time:
- Prep & Cook Time: 20 minutes

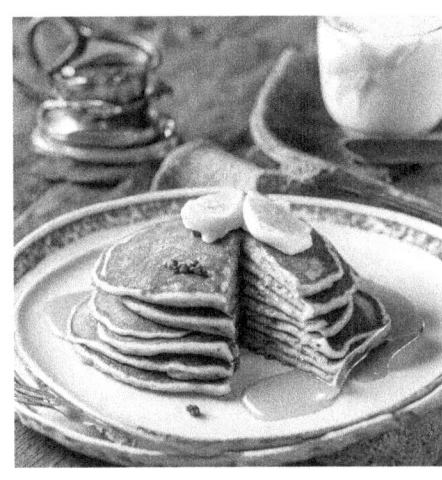

12. Muesli

Ingredients:
- 2 cups rolled oats
- 1/2 cup sliced almonds
- 1/2 cup dried cranberries or raisins
- 2 tablespoons pumpkin seeds
- 1 teaspoon cinnamon
- Milk or yogurt, for serving
- Fresh fruits, for topping

Instructions:
1. In a large mixing bowl, combine the oats, almonds, dried cranberries or raisins, pumpkin seeds, and cinnamon.
2. Store the muesli in an airtight container.
3. To serve, scoop the desired amount of muesli into a bowl and top with milk or yogurt and fresh fruits.

Serves:
- 6 servings

Nutritional Info (per serving, without milk/yogurt and fruits):
- Calories: 300
- Protein: 10g
- Carbohydrates: 45g
- Fat: 10g
- Fiber: 7g
- Calcium: 60mg

Cooking Time:
- Prep Time: 10 minutes (plus overnight soaking if preferred)

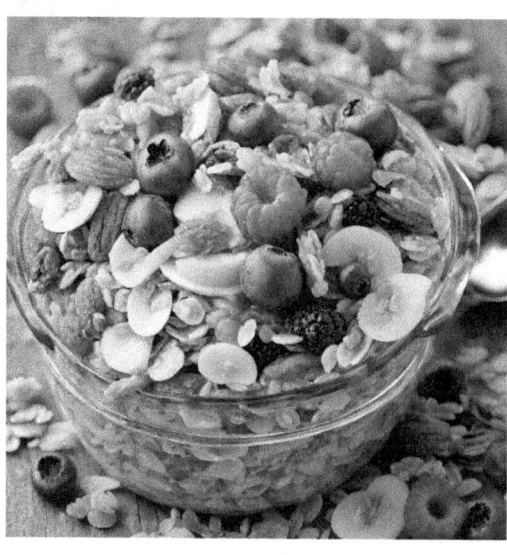

13. Melon Salad

Ingredients:
- 2 cups cubed cantaloupe
- 2 cups cubed honeydew melon
- 1 cup watermelon cubes
- 2 tablespoons fresh mint, chopped
- Juice of 1 lime
- 1 tablespoon honey (optional)

Instructions:
1. In a large bowl, combine the cantaloupe, honeydew, and watermelon cubes.
2. Add the chopped fresh mint.
3. In a small bowl, whisk together the lime juice and honey until well combined.
4. Pour the dressing over the melon mixture and toss gently to coat.
5. Chill in the refrigerator for at least 1 hour before serving.

Serves:
- 4 servings

Nutritional Info (per serving):
- Calories: 90
- Protein: 1.5g
- Carbohydrates: 22g
- Fat: 0.5g
- Fiber: 1.5g
- Calcium: 15mg

Cooking Time:
- Prep Time: 15 minutes (plus chilling time)

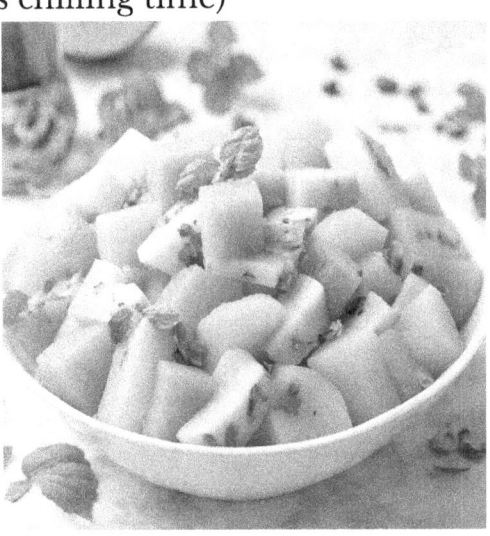

14. Zucchini Bread
Ingredients:
- 1 1/2 cups whole wheat flour
- 1/2 teaspoon salt
- 1/2 teaspoon baking soda
- 1/2 teaspoon baking powder
- 1 1/2 teaspoons cinnamon
- 1/4 cup unsweetened applesauce
- 1/2 cup honey or maple syrup
- 1 egg
- 1 teaspoon vanilla extract
- 1 cup grated zucchini (water squeezed out)
- 1/2 cup chopped walnuts (optional)

Instructions:
1. Preheat the oven to 350°F (175°C) and grease a 9x5 inch loaf pan.
2. In a bowl, combine the flour, salt, baking soda, baking powder, and cinnamon.
3. In a separate bowl, mix the applesauce, honey, egg, and vanilla.
4. Stir the wet ingredients into the dry ingredients, then fold in the zucchini (and walnuts, if using).
5. Pour the batter into the prepared loaf pan.
6. Bake for 50-60 minutes, or until a toothpick inserted into the center comes out clean.
7. Allow to cool in the pan for 10 minutes, then transfer to a wire rack to cool completely.

Serves:
- 10 servings

Nutritional Info (per serving):
- Calories: 160
- Protein: 3g
- Carbohydrates: 32g
- Fat: 3g (without walnuts)
- Fiber: 3g
- Calcium: 30mg

Cooking Time:
- Prep Time: 15 minutes; Bake Time: 50-60 minutes

15. Scrambled Tofu

Ingredients:
- 1 block (14 oz) firm tofu, drained and crumbled
- 1 tablespoon olive oil
- 1/2 onion, finely chopped
- 1/2 bell pepper, chopped
- 1 teaspoon turmeric
- 1/2 teaspoon garlic powder
- Salt and pepper to taste
- 2 tablespoons nutritional yeast (optional)
- Fresh herbs (e.g., parsley, chives), for garnish

Instructions:
1. Heat the olive oil in a non-stick skillet over medium heat.
2. Add the onion and bell pepper, sautéing until softened.
3. Add the crumbled tofu, turmeric, garlic powder, salt, and pepper.
4. Cook, stirring frequently, until the tofu is heated through and begins to brown slightly, about 5-7 minutes.
5. Stir in the nutritional yeast, if using, and cook for another minute.
6. Garnish with fresh herbs before serving.

Serves:
- 2-3 servings

Nutritional Info (per serving):
- Calories: 200
- Protein: 18g
- Carbohydrates: 7g
- Fat: 12g
- Fiber: 2g
- Calcium: 150mg

Cooking Time:
- Prep & Cook Time: 15 minutes

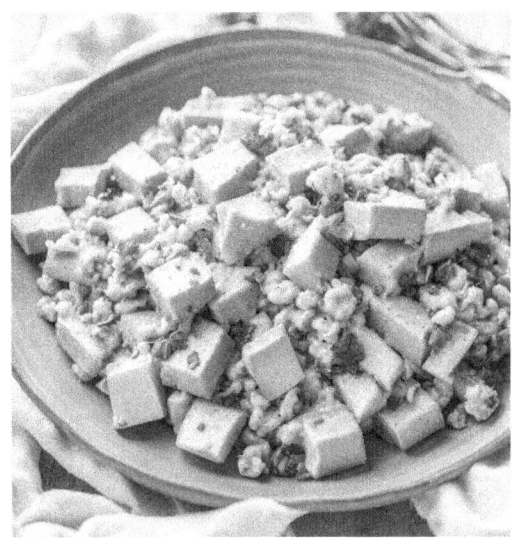

16. Rice Pudding

Ingredients:
- 1 cup cooked white rice
- 2 cups milk (or almond milk)
- 1/3 cup sugar
- 1/4 teaspoon salt
- 1/2 teaspoon vanilla extract
- 1/4 teaspoon cinnamon
- 1/4 cup raisins (optional)

Instructions:
1. In a saucepan, combine the cooked rice, milk, sugar, and salt.
2. Cook over medium heat, stirring occasionally, until thick and creamy.
3. Remove from heat and stir in vanilla extract, cinnamon, and raisins.
4. Pour the pudding into serving dishes.
5. Serve warm or chilled.

Serves:
- 4 servings

Nutrition:
- Calories:
- Protein:
- Carbo
- Fat: 2g
- Fiber:
- Calcium

Cooking
- Prep &

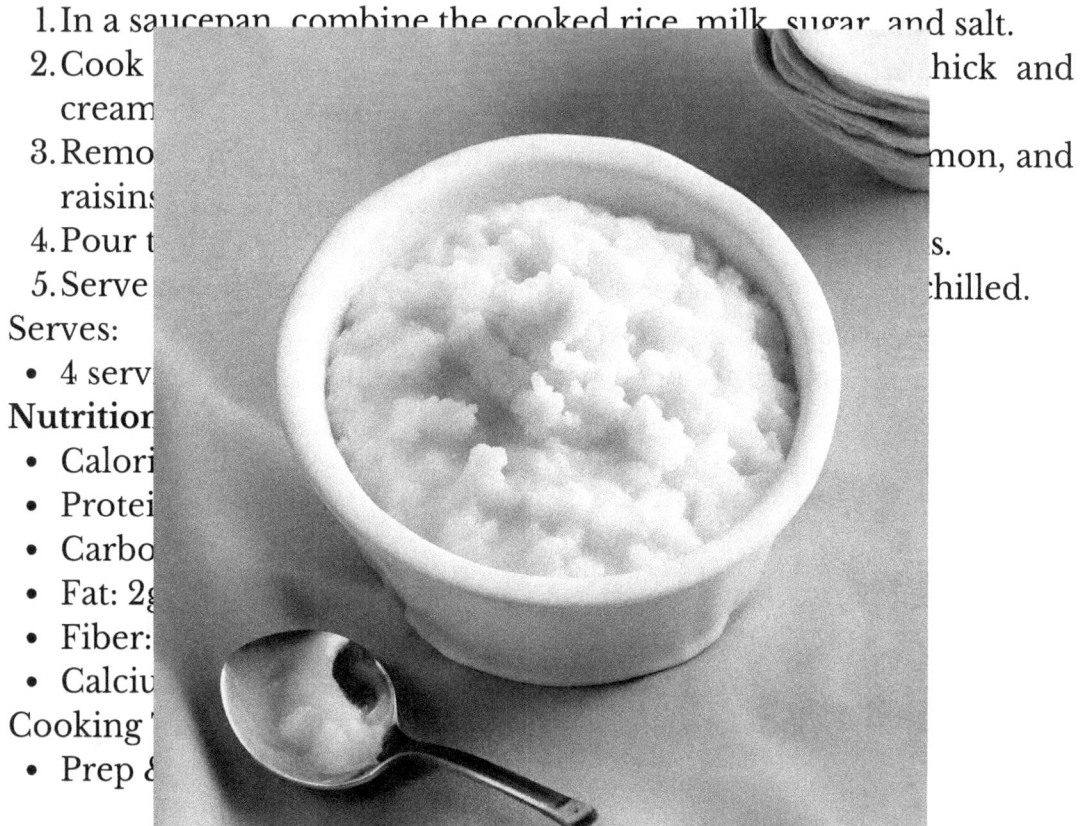

17. Polenta

Ingredients:
- 1 cup polenta (cornmeal)
- 4 cups water or vegetable broth
- 1/2 teaspoon salt
- 2 tablespoons butter or olive oil
- 1/4 cup grated Parmesan cheese (optional)

Instructions:
1. In a large saucepan, bring the water or broth to a boil.
2. Gradually whisk in the polenta and salt, reducing the heat to low.
3. Continue to cook, stirring constantly, until the polenta thickens and pulls away from the sides of the pan, about 20-30 minutes.
4. Remove from heat and stir in the butter and Parmesan cheese until well incorporated.
5. Serve hot, either soft or poured into a greased pan to cool and solidify, then sliced.

Serves:
- 4 servings

Nutritional Info (per serving):
- Calories: 200
- Protein: 4g
- Carbohydrates: 38g
- Fat: 4g (with olive oil)
- Fiber: 2g
- Calcium: 20mg

Cooking Time:
- Prep & Cook Time: 35 minutes

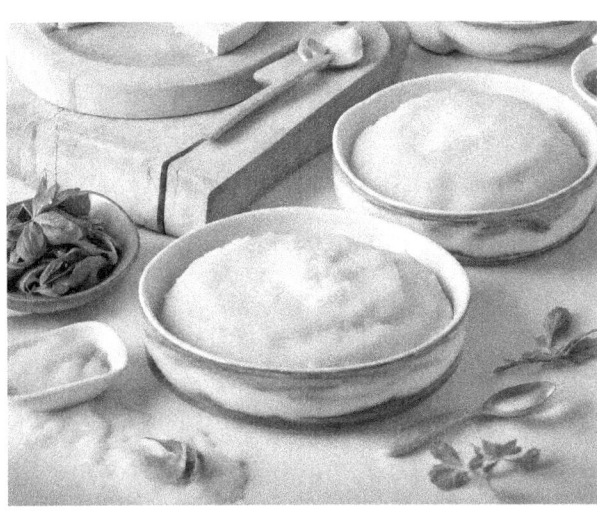

18. Shakshuka

Ingredients:
- 1 tablespoon olive oil
- 1 large onion, chopped
- 1 red bell pepper, chopped
- 2 garlic cloves, minced
- 1 teaspoon paprika
- 1 teaspoon cumin
- 1 can (28 oz) whole peeled tomatoes
- Salt and pepper to taste
- 4-6 large eggs
- Fresh parsley, for garnish

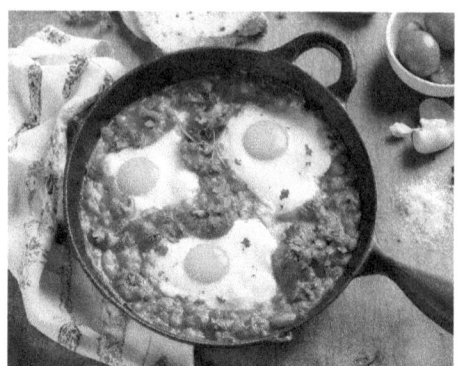

Instructions:
1. Heat the olive oil in a large skillet over medium heat.
2. Add the onion and bell pepper, sautéing until softened.
3. Stir in the garlic, paprika, and cumin, cooking for another minute.
4. Pour in the tomatoes (break them down as you stir) and season with salt and pepper. Simmer for 10-15 minutes to allow flavors to meld.
5. Make wells in the sauce and crack an egg into each. Cover the skillet and cook until the eggs are done to your liking.
6. Garnish with fresh parsley and serve directly from the skillet.

Serves:
- 4-6 servings

Nutritional Info (per serving for 4 servings):
- Calories: 220
- Protein: 12g
- Carbohydrates: 18g
- Fat: 12g
- Fiber: 4g
- Calcium: 80mg

Cooking Time:
- Prep & Cook Time: 30 minutes

19. Sweet Potato Hash

Ingredients:
- 2 large sweet potatoes, peeled and diced
- 1 tablespoon olive oil
- 1 onion, diced
- 1 red bell pepper, diced
- 2 cloves garlic, minced
- 1/2 teaspoon smoked paprika
- Salt and pepper to taste
- 4 eggs (optional)
- Fresh parsley, for garnish

Instructions:
1. Heat the olive oil in a large skillet over medium heat.
2. Add the sweet potatoes, onion, and bell pepper. Cook, stirring occasionally, until the vegetables are tender and beginning to brown, about 10-15 minutes.
3. Stir in the garlic, smoked paprika, salt, and pepper, cooking for another 2 minutes.
4. If using eggs, make wells in the hash and crack an egg into each. Cover and cook until the eggs are set to your liking.
5. Garnish with fresh parsley and serve hot.

Serves:
- 4 servings

Nutritional Info (per serving):
- Calories: 250 (without eggs)
- Protein: 5g
- Carbohydrates: 37g
- Fat: 9g
- Fiber: 6g
- Calcium: 60mg

Cooking Time:
- Prep & Cook Time: 30 minutes

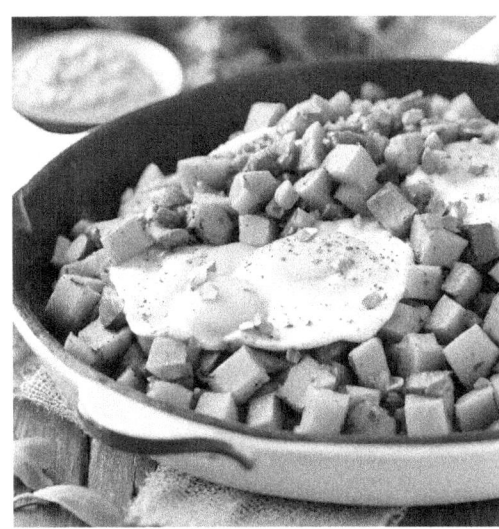

20. Veggie Breakfast Tacos

Ingredients:
- 4 small corn tortillas
- 1 cup scrambled eggs (about 4 eggs)
- 1/2 cup black beans, rinsed and drained
- 1 avocado, sliced
- 1/2 cup diced tomatoes
- 1/4 cup shredded low-fat cheese
- 2 tablespoons chopped cilantro
- Lime wedges for serving

Instructions:
1. Warm the tortillas in a dry skillet or on a grill.
2. Divide the scrambled eggs evenly among the tortillas.
3. Top each with black beans, avocado slices, diced tomatoes, and shredded cheese.
4. Garnish with chopped cilantro and serve with a lime wedge on the side.

Serves:
- 4 servings (1 taco each)

Nutritional Info (per serving):
- Calories: 300
- Protein: 15g
- Carbohydrates: 30g
- Fat: 15g
- Fiber: 7g
- Calcium: 150mg

Cooking Time:
- Prep & Cook Time: 20 minutes

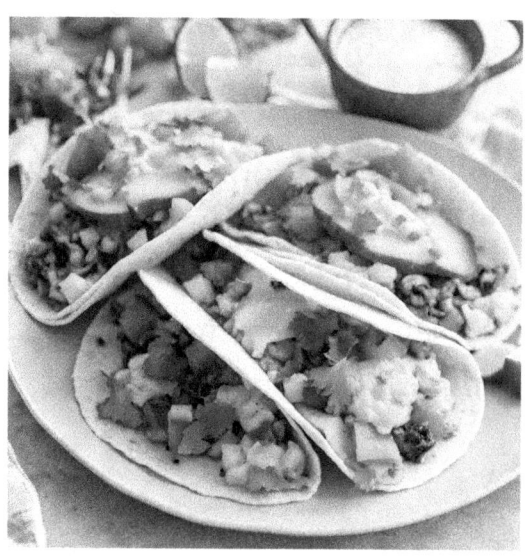

21. Pear and Walnut Oatmeal

Ingredients:
- 1 cup rolled oats
- 2 cups water or milk
- 1 ripe pear, diced
- 1/4 cup chopped walnuts
- 1/2 teaspoon cinnamon
- 1 tablespoon honey or maple syrup

Instructions:
1. Combine oats and water (or milk) in a saucepan and bring to a boil.
2. Reduce _____ until oats are so_____
3. Stir i_____ cook for anoth_____
4. Sweet_____

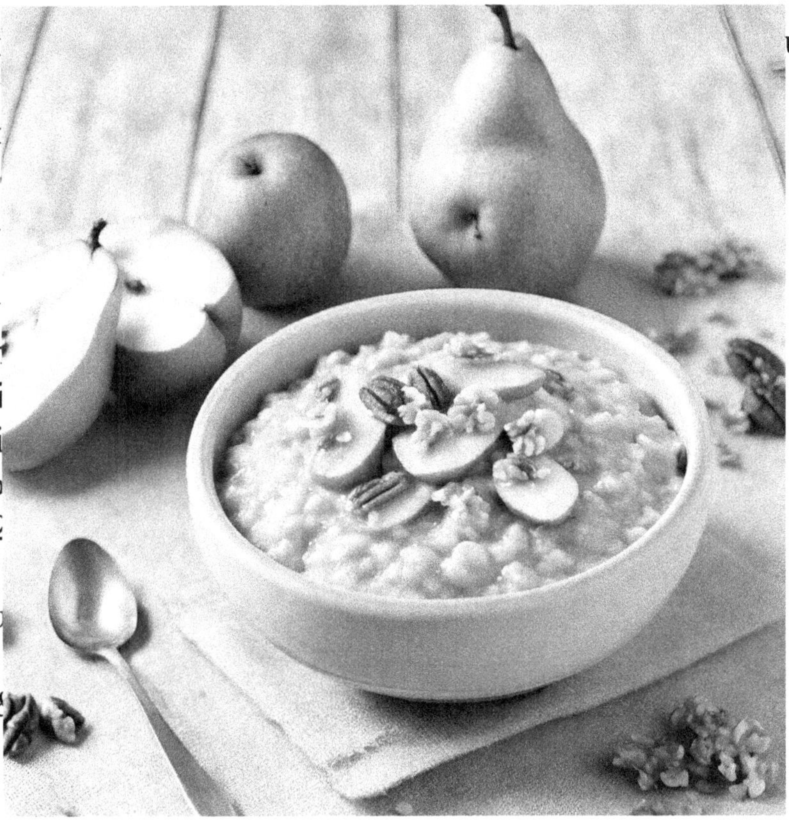

Serves:
- 2 serv_____

Nutrition
- Calori_____
- Protei_____
- Carbo_____
- Fat: 1_____
- Fiber:_____
- Calciu_____

Cooking
- Prep &_____

22. Apple Cinnamon Quinoa Bowl

Ingredients:
- 1 cup quinoa, rinsed
- 2 cups water
- 1 apple, diced
- 1/2 teaspoon cinnamon
- 2 tablespoons maple syrup
- 1/4 cup chopped almonds

Instructions:
1. Combine quinoa and water in a saucepan. Bring to a boil, then cover and reduce to a simmer for 15 minutes, or until all water is absorbed.
2. Remove from heat and let it sit covered for 5 minutes. Fluff with a fork.
3. Stir in the diced apple, cinnamon, and maple syrup.
4. Top with chopped almonds before serving.

Serves:
- 2 servings

Nutritional Info (per serving):
- Calories: 350
- Protein: 8g
- Carbohydrates: 65g
- Fat: 7g
- Fiber: 8g
- Calcium: 40mg

Cooking Time:
- Prep & Cook Time: 25 minutes

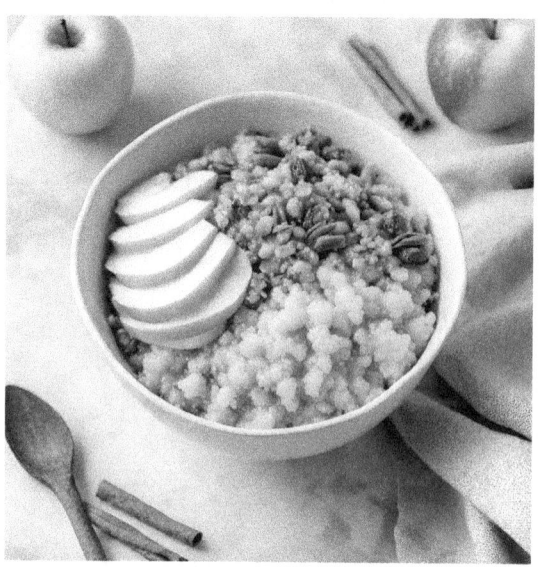

23. Pumpkin Seed Granola

Ingredients:
- 2 cups rolled oats
- 1 cup raw pumpkin seeds
- 1/2 cup maple syrup
- 1/4 cup coconut oil, melted
- 1 teaspoon vanilla extract
- 1/2 teaspoon salt
- 1/2 teaspoon cinnamon

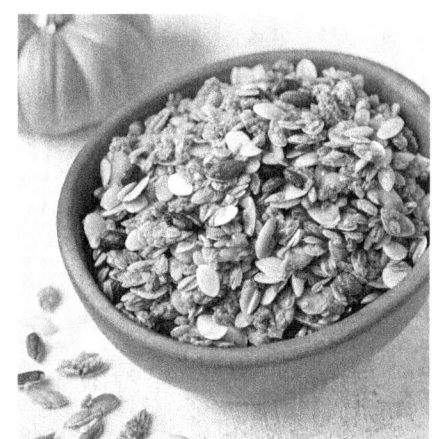

Instructions:
1. Preheat the oven to 300°F (150°C) and line a baking sheet with parchment paper.
2. In a large bowl, mix oats, pumpkin seeds, cinnamon, and salt.
3. In a separate bowl, whisk together maple syrup, melted coconut oil, and vanilla.
4. Combine both mixtures and spread evenly on the prepared baking sheet.
5. Bake for 30-40 minutes, stirring occasionally, until golden brown.
6. Let it cool completely before storing in an airtight container.

Serves:
- 8 servings

Nutritional Info (per serving):
- Calories: 300
- Protein: 7g
- Carbohydrates: 30g
- Fat: 18g
- Fiber: 4g
- Calcium: 20mg

Cooking Time:
- Prep Time: 10 minutes; Bake Time: 30-40 minutes

24. Cornmeal Porridge

Instructions:
1. In a large saucepan, bring the water to a boil and add the salt.
2. Gradually whisk in the cornmeal, ensuring there are no lumps.
3. Reduce the heat to low and simmer, stirring constantly, until the mixture thickens and the cornmeal is cooked through, about 10-15 minutes.
4. Stir in the milk, sugar (or honey), and cinnamon. Cook for another 2-3 minutes, stirring frequently.
5. Serve warm, adjusting the sweetness or milk to your preference.

Serves:
- 4 serv

Nutrition
- Calori
- Protei
- Carbo
- Fat: 2.
- Fiber:
- Calciu

Cooking
- Prep &

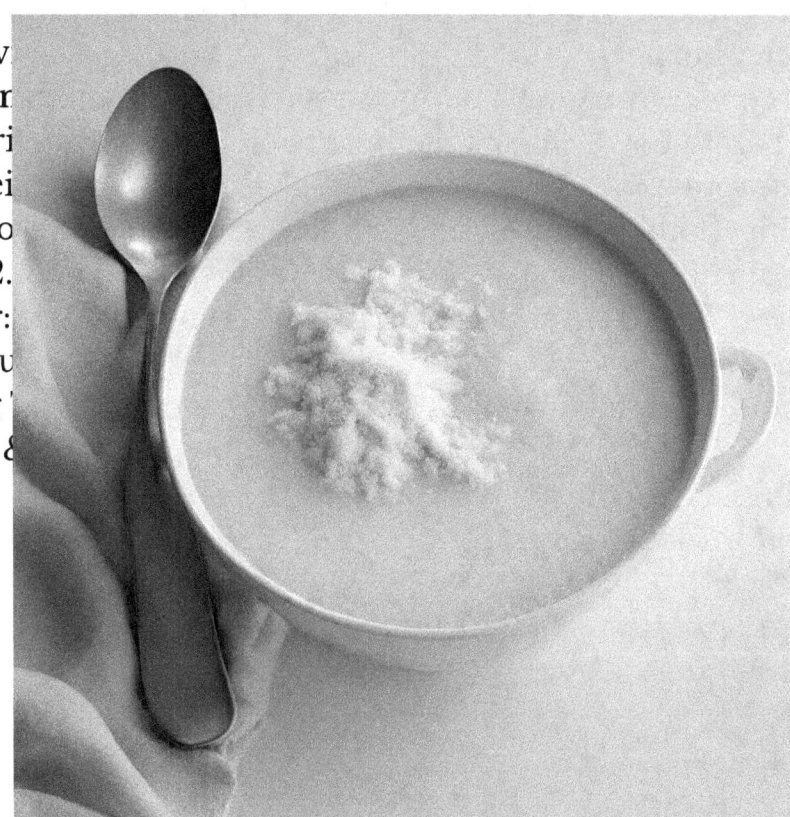

25. Almond Flour Biscuits

Ingredients:
- 2 cups almond flour
- 1 teaspoon baking powder
- 1/2 teaspoon salt
- 2 tablespoons cold butter, diced (or coconut oil for a dairy-free option)
- 2 eggs, beaten
- 1/3 cup almond milk

Instructions:
1. Preheat the oven to 350°F (175°C) and line a baking sheet with parch
2. In a b
3. Cut in
4. Stir in
5. Drop
   out ar
6. Bake f

Serves:
- 8 bisc

Nutrition
- Calori
- Protei
- Carbo
- Fat: 16
- Fiber:
- Calciu

Cooking
- Prep

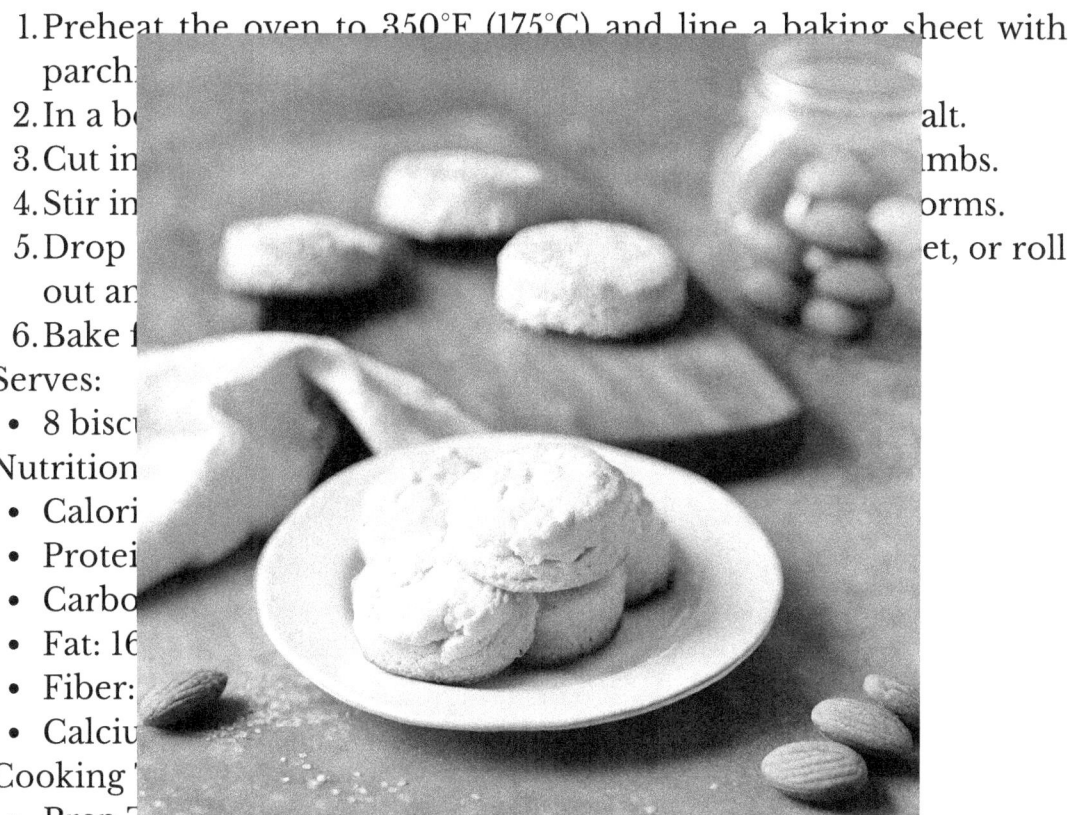

26. Berry and Flaxseed Smoothie

Ingredients:
- 1 cup mixed berries (fresh or frozen)
- 1 banana
- 1 tablespoon ground flaxseed
- 1 cup spinach (optional)
- 1 cup almond milk or water
- 1 tablespoon honey or maple syrup (optional)

Instructions:
1. Place the mixed berries, banana, ground flaxseed, spinach (if using), and almond milk (or water) in a blender.
2. Blend on high until smooth. Add honey or maple syrup to sweeten, if desired.
3. Taste and adjust the sweetness or liquid as needed. Blend again if necessary.
4. Serve immediately, or refrigerate for up to 24 hours.

Serves:
- 2 servings

Nutritional Info (per serving):
- Calories: 150
- Protein: 3g
- Carbohydrates: 30g
- Fat: 3g
- Fiber: 5g
- Calcium: 150mg (if using fortified almond milk)

Cooking Time:
- Prep & Blend Time: 5 minutes

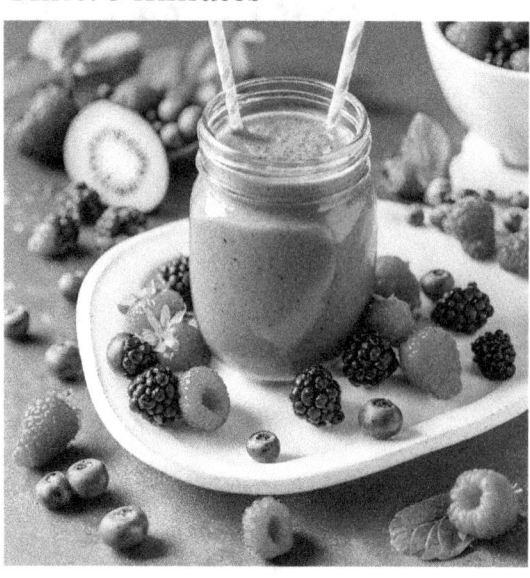

Lunch Recipes

1. Grilled Chicken Salad
Ingredients:
- 2 boneless, skinless chicken breasts
- 1 tablespoon olive oil
- Salt and pepper to taste
- 4 cups mixed salad greens
- 1 cup cherry tomatoes, halved
- 1 cucumber, sliced
- 1/4 cup sliced red onion
- 1/4 cup balsamic vinaigrette dressing

Instructions:
1. Preheat the grill to medium-high heat.
2. Brush the chicken breasts with olive oil and season with salt and pepper.
3. Grill the chicken for 6-7 minutes per side or until fully cooked (internal temperature of 165°F/74°C).
4. Let the chicken rest for 5 minutes, then slice thinly.
5. In a large salad bowl, toss the mixed greens, cherry tomatoes, cucumber, and red onion.
6. Top the salad with the sliced chicken and drizzle with balsamic vinaigrette.

Serves:
- 4 servings

Nutritional Info (per serving):
- Calories: 250
- Protein: 26g
- Carbohydrates: 10g
- Fat: 12g
- Fiber: 2g
- Calcium: 50mg

Cooking Time:
- Prep & Cook Time: 20 minutes

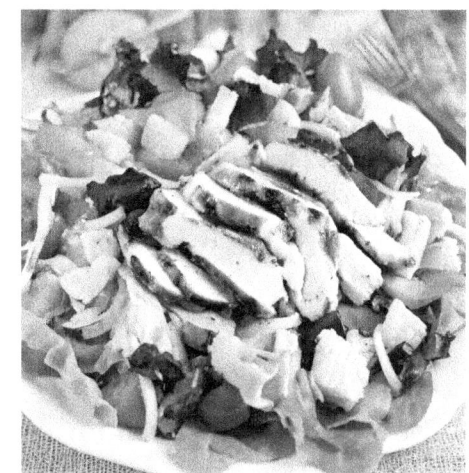

2. Lentil Soup

Ingredients:

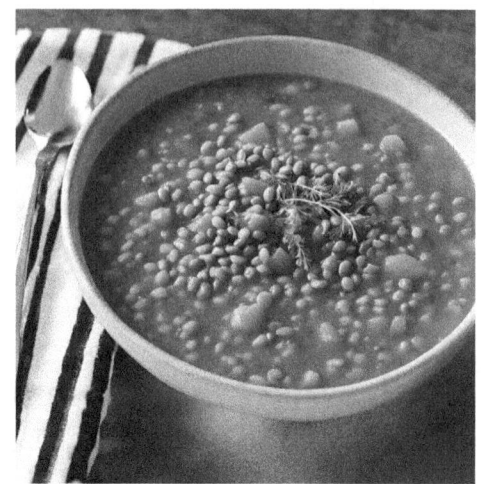

- 1 tablespoon olive oil
- 1 onion, diced
- 2 carrots, peeled and diced
- 2 celery stalks, diced
- 2 garlic cloves, minced
- 1 cup dried lentils, rinsed
- 6 cups vegetable broth
- 1 teaspoon ground cumin
- Salt and pepper to taste
- 2 tablespoons chopped fresh parsley

Instructions:

1. Heat the olive oil in a large pot over medium heat.
2. Add the onion, carrots, celery, and garlic. Cook until the vegetables are softened, about 5 minutes.
3. Stir in the lentils, vegetable broth, and cumin. Season with salt and pepper.
4. Bring to a boil, then reduce the heat and simmer, covered, for about 30 minutes, or until the lentils are tender.
5. Puree part of the soup with an immersion blender for a thicker consistency if desired.
6. Stir in the parsley before serving.

Serves:

- 6 servings

Nutritional Info (per serving):

- Calories: 200
- Protein: 12g
- Carbohydrates: 30g
- Fat: 3g
- Fiber: 15g
- Calcium: 40mg

Cooking Time:

- Prep & Cook Time: 45 minutes

3. Quinoa Stuffed Bell Peppers

Ingredients:
- 4 large bell peppers, halved and seeded
- 1 cup quinoa, cooked
- 1 tablespoon olive oil
- 1/2 onion, diced
- 2 garlic cloves, minced
- 1 cup spinach, chopped
- 1 tomato, diced
- 1/2 cup corn (fresh or frozen)
- 1 teaspoon cumin
- Salt and pepper to taste
- 1/2 cup shredded low-fat cheese (optional)

Instructions:
1. Preheat the oven to 375°F (190°C).
2. Place the bell pepper halves in a baking dish, cut-side up.
3. Heat the olive oil in a skillet over medium heat. Add the onion and garlic, sautéing until softened.
4. Stir in the spinach, tomato, corn, and cumin. Cook until the spinach is wilted.
5. Mix the cooked quinoa into the skillet and season with salt and pepper.
6. Spoon the quinoa mixture into each bell pepper half.
7. Top with shredded cheese if desired.
8. Cover with foil and bake for 30 minutes. Uncover and bake for an additional 10 minutes or until the peppers are tender.

Serves:
- 4 servings

Nutritional Info (per serving):
- Calories: 250
- Protein: 10g
- Carbohydrates: 40g
- Fat: 7g
- Fiber: 7g
- Calcium: 100mg (if adding cheese)

Cooking Time:
- Prep & Cook Time: 50 minutes

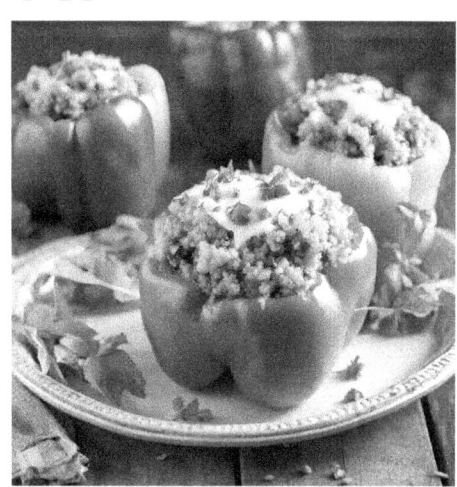

4. Turkey Wrap

Ingredients:
- 4 whole wheat tortillas
- 8 slices turkey breast (low sodium)
- 1 cup mixed salad greens
- 1 tomato, sliced
- 1/4 cup low-fat mayonnaise or Greek yogurt
- 1 avocado, sliced
- Salt and pepper to taste

Instructions:
1. Spread each tortilla evenly with low-fat mayonnaise or Greek yogurt.
2. Place two slices of turkey breast on each tortilla.
3. Add a layer of mixed salad greens and tomato slices.
4. Top with avocado slices and season with salt and pepper.
5. Roll up the tortillas tightly, cut in half, and serve.

Serves:
- 4 servings

Nutritional Info (per serving):
- Calories: 300
- Protein: 20g
- Carbohydrates: 35g
- Fat: 10g
- Fiber: 5g
- Calcium: 40mg

Cooking Time:
- Prep Time: 15 minutes

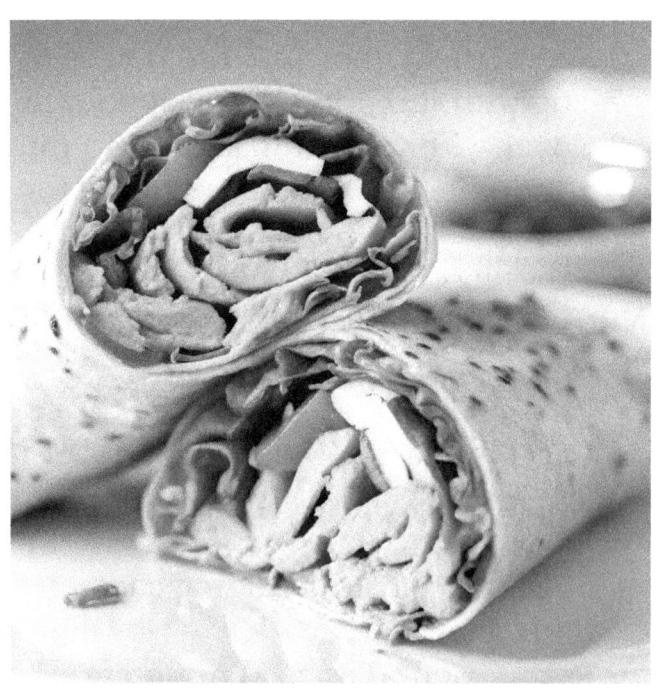

5. Vegetarian Chili
Ingredients:
- 1 tablespoon olive oil
- 1 onion, chopped
- 2 garlic cloves, minced
- 1 bell pepper, chopped
- 2 carrots, diced
- 2 celery stalks, diced
- 1 zucchini, diced
- 1 can (15 oz) black beans, drained and rinsed
- 1 can (15 oz) kidney beans, drained and rinsed
- 1 can (
- 2 table
- 1 teasp
- 1 teasp
- Salt a
- Fresh

Instructi
1. Heat t
2. Add   onion is transl
3. Add t   king until they b
4. Stir i   oes, chili powd   er.
5. Bring   simmer, uncov
6. Adjust   ith fresh cilantr

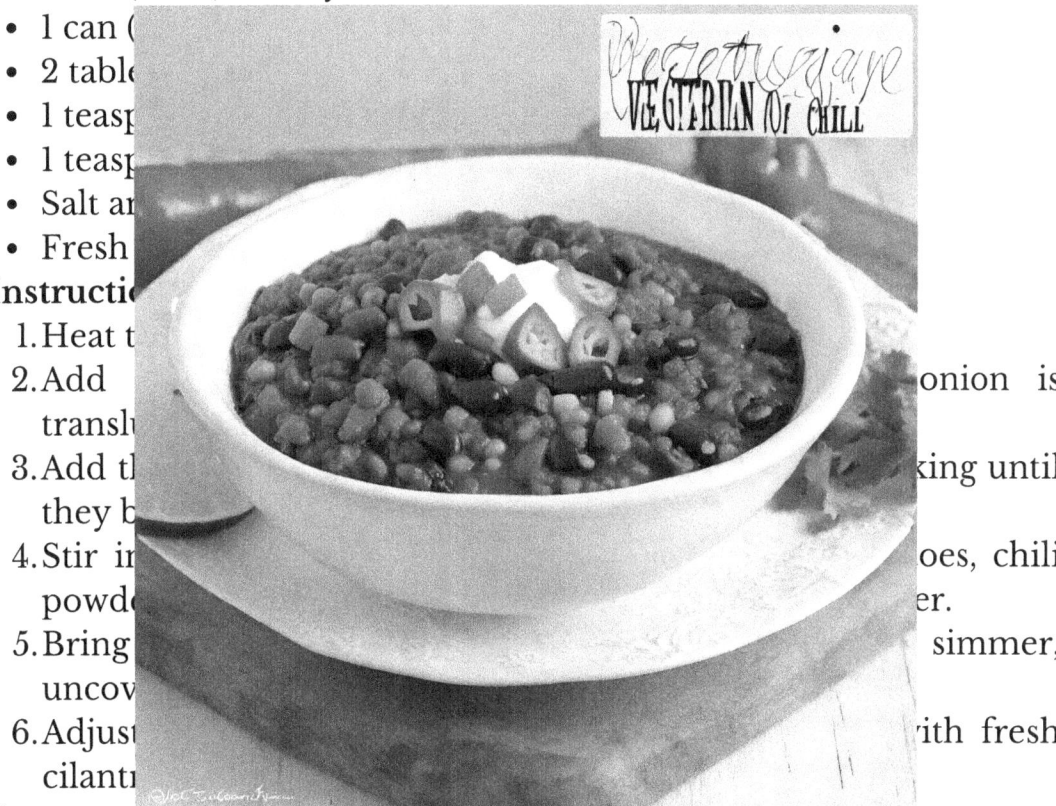

Serves:
- 6 servings

Nutritional Info (per serving):
- Calories: 250 Protein: 12g
- Carbohydrates: 45g
- Fat: 4g
- Fiber: 15g
- Calcium: 80mg

Cooking Time:
- Prep & Cook Time: 45 minutes

6. Salmon and Arugula Salad

Ingredients:
- 4 salmon fillets (4 oz each)
- 2 tablespoons olive oil
- Salt and pepper to taste
- 4 cups arugula
- 1 cup cherry tomatoes, halved
- 1/4 red onion, thinly sliced
- 2 tablespoons balsamic vinegar
- 1 tablespoon honey
- 1 tablespoon Dijon mustard

Instructions:
1. Prehe
2. Brush   season with s
3. Grill   cooked throu
4. In a   nd red onion
5. Whisk   honey, and D
6. Divide   on, and drizzl

Serves:
- 4 serv

Nutrition
- Calori
- Protei
- Carbo
- Fat: 19g
- Fiber: 1g
- Calcium: 60mg

Cooking Time:
- Prep & Cook Time: 20 minutes

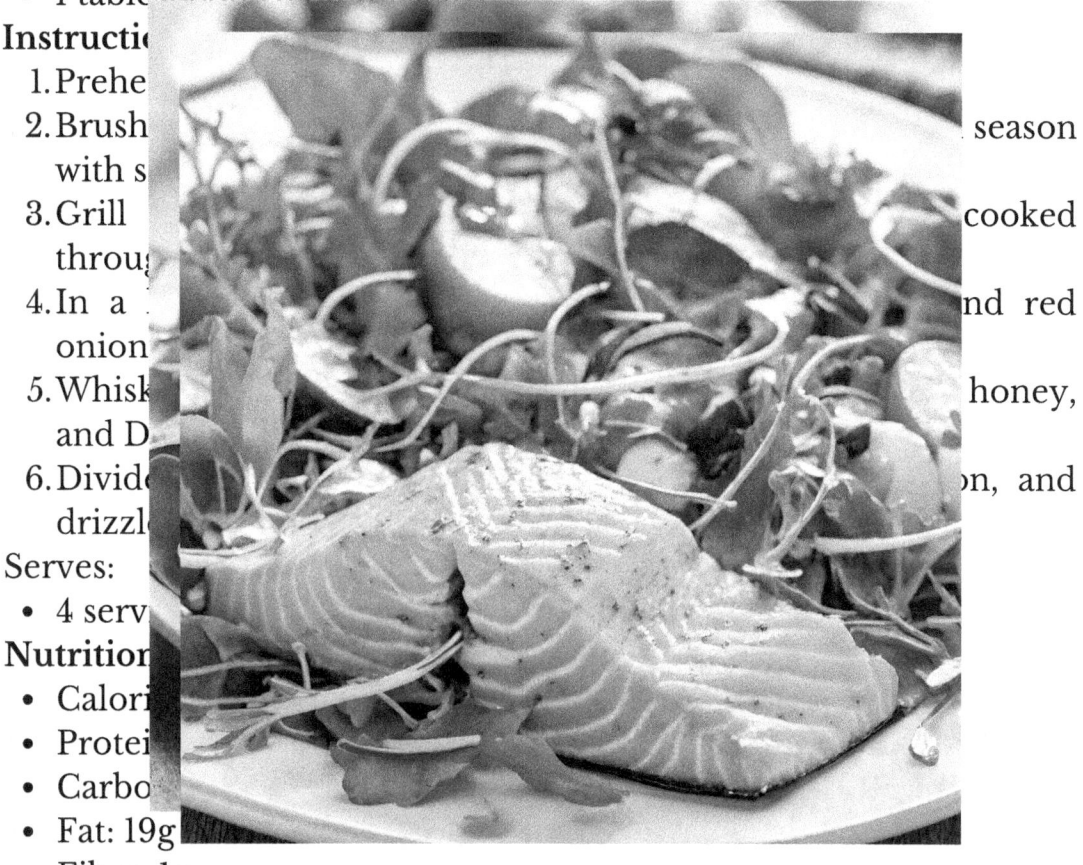

7. Roasted Vegetable Plate

Ingredients:
- 2 bell peppers, sliced
- 2 zucchinis, sliced
- 1 eggplant, sliced
- 2 tablespoons olive oil
- Salt and pepper to taste
- 1 teaspoon dried thyme

Instructions:
1. Preheat the oven to 400°F (200°C).
2. Arrange the sliced vegetables on a baking sheet.
3. Drizzle with olive oil and season with salt, pepper, and thyme.
4. Roast in the oven for 25-30 minutes, or until vegetables are tender and slightly caramelized.

Serves:
- 4 servings

Nutritional Info (per serving):
- Calories: 150
- Protein: 3g
- Carbohydrates: 18g
- Fat: 9g
- Fiber: 6g
- Calcium: 30mg

Cooking Time:
- Prep & Cook Time: 35 minutes

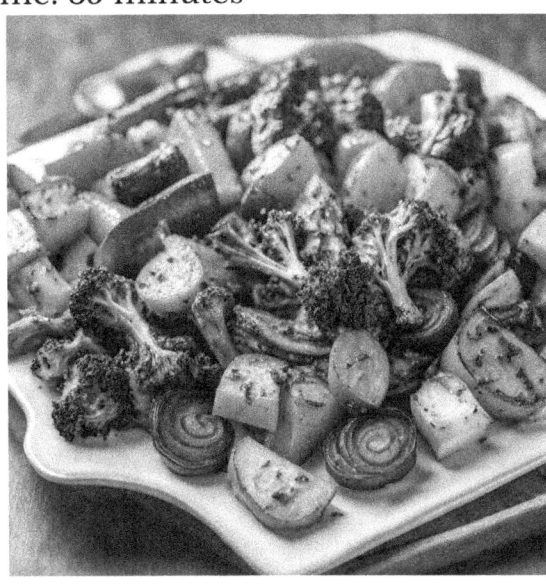

8. Pasta Primavera

Ingredients:
- 8 oz whole wheat pasta
- 2 tablespoons olive oil
- 1 zucchini, sliced
- 1 bell pepper, sliced
- 1/2 cup cherry tomatoes, halved
- 1/4 cup peas
- 2 garlic cloves, minced
- Salt and pepper to taste
- 1/4 cup grated Parmesan cheese
- 1 tablespoon fresh basil, chopped

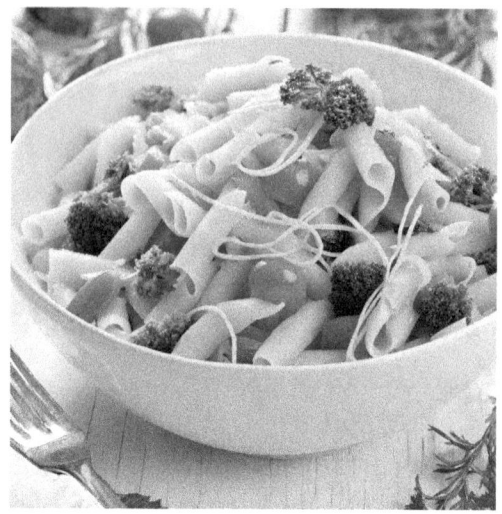

Instructions:
1. Cook the pasta according to package instructions; drain and set aside.
2. In a large skillet, heat the olive oil over medium heat.
3. Add the zucchini, bell pepper, cherry tomatoes, peas, and garlic. Sauté until the vegetables are tender.
4. Toss the cooked pasta with the sautéed vegetables, season with salt and pepper.
5. Serve sprinkled with Parmesan cheese and fresh basil.

Serves:
- 4 servings

Nutritional Info (per serving):
- Calories: 320
- Protein: 12g
- Carbohydrates: 48g
- Fat: 10g
- Fiber: 8g
- Calcium: 100mg

Cooking Time:
- Prep & Cook Time: 30 minutes

9. Tofu Stir-Fry

Ingredients:
- 1 block (14 oz) firm tofu, drained and cubed
- 2 tablespoons soy sauce
- 1 tablespoon sesame oil
- 2 cups mixed vegetables (bell peppers, broccoli, carrots)
- 1 garlic clove, minced
- 1 teaspoon ginger, minced
- 2 tablespoons vegetable broth or water
- 1 tablespoon cornstarch mixed with 2 tablespoons water (optional for thickening)

Instructions:
1. Marinate the tofu cubes in soy sauce for at least 10 minutes.
2. Heat the sesame oil in a large skillet or wok over medium-high heat.
3. Add the tofu and stir-fry until golden brown, then remove and set aside.
4. In the same skillet, add the mixed vegetables, garlic, and ginger. Stir-fry until vegetables are just tender.
5. Return the tofu to the skillet, add the vegetable broth, and bring to a simmer.
6. If a thicker sauce is desired, add the cornstarch-water mixture and cook until thickened.
7. Serve hot, ideally over rice or quinoa.

Serves:
- 4 servings

Nutritional Info (per serving):
- Calories: 200
- Protein: 12g
- Carbohydrates: 10g
- Fat: 12g
- Fiber: 3g
- Calcium: 150mg

Cooking Time:
- Prep & Cook Time: 30 minutes

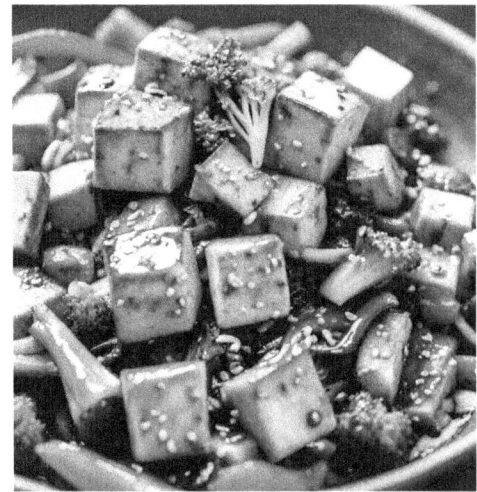

10. Vegetable Curry

Ingredients:
- 1 tablespoon coconut oil
- 1 onion, diced
- 2 garlic cloves, minced
- 1 tablespoon curry powder
- 1 teaspoon ground turmeric
- 1 can (14 oz) coconut milk
- 2 cups cauliflower florets
- 1 bell pepper, chopped
- 1 zucchini, chopped
- 1 carrot
- Salt to
- Fresh

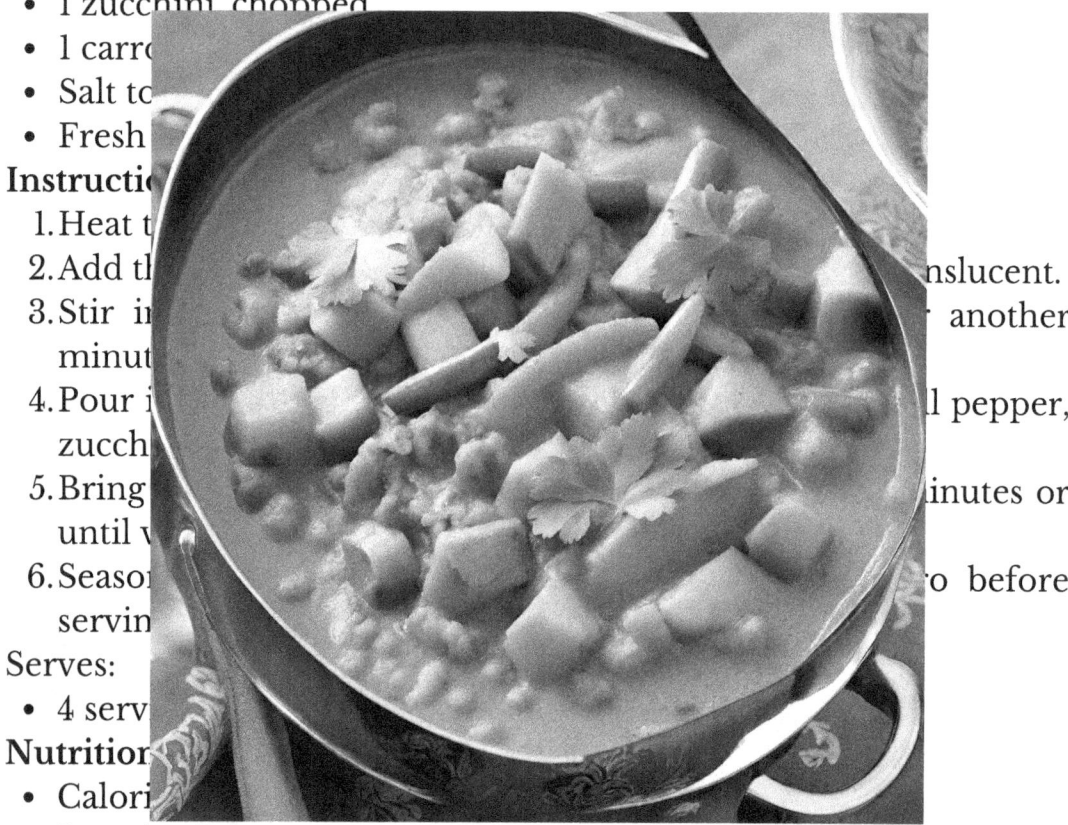

Instructions:
1. Heat t
2. Add t... nslucent.
3. Stir i... another minut
4. Pour i... l pepper, zucch
5. Bring ... inutes or until
6. Season ... o before servin

Serves:
- 4 serv

Nutrition
- Calori
- Protein: 5g
- Carbohydrates: 15g
- Fat: 22g
- Fiber: 4g
- Calcium: 40mg

Cooking Time:
- Prep & Cook Time: 30 minutes

11. Egg Salad

Ingredients:
- 8 hard-boiled eggs, peeled and chopped
- 1/4 cup mayonnaise (low-fat or avocado-based)
- 2 tablespoons mustard
- Salt and pepper to taste
- 1/4 cup chopped celery
- 1 tablespoon chopped fresh chives

Instructions:
1. In a bowl, combine the chopped eggs, mayonnaise, mustard, salt, and pepper.
2. Stir in the celery and chives.
3. Adjust seasoning if necessary and chill until serving.

Serves:
- 4 servings

Nutritional Info (per serving):
- Calories: 210
- Protein: 13g
- Carbohydrates: 2g
- Fat: 16g
- Fiber: 0g
- Calcium: 50mg

Cooking Time:
- Prep Time: 10 minutes (additional time for boiling eggs)

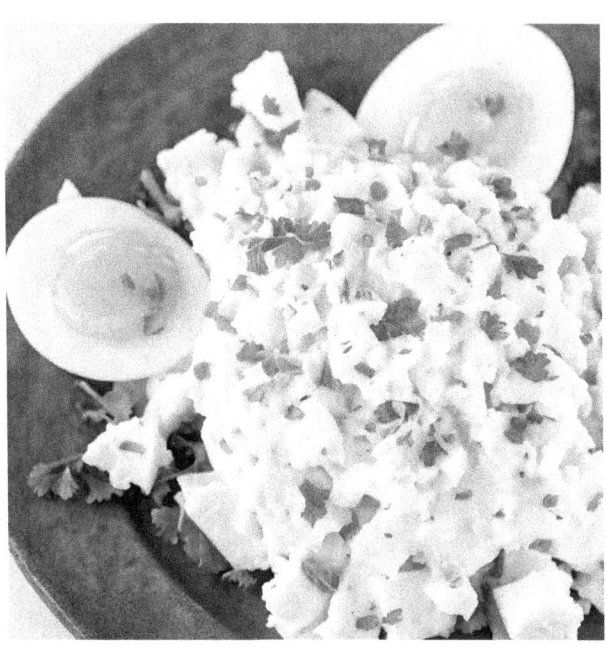

12. Shrimp and Avocado Salad

Ingredients:
- 1 lb cooked shrimp, peeled and deveined
- 2 avocados, diced
- 1 cup cherry tomatoes, halved
- 1/4 cup red onion, finely chopped
- Juice of 1 lime
- 2 tablespoons olive oil
- Salt and pepper to taste
- Fresh cilantro, chopped (optional)

Instructions:
1. In a large bowl, combine the shrimp, avocados, cherry tomatoes, and red onion.
2. Drizzle with lime juice and olive oil. Gently toss to combine.
3. Season with salt and pepper, and garnish with cilantro if desired.
4. Serve immediately or chill until ready to serve.

Serves:
- 4 servings

Nutritional Info (per serving):
- Calories: 290
- Protein: 24g
- Carbohydrates: 12g
- Fat: 18g
- Fiber: 6g
- Calcium: 150mg

Cooking Time:
- Prep Time: 15 minutes

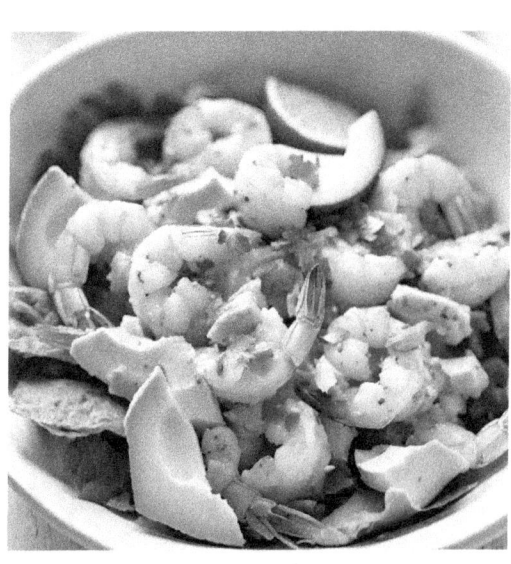

13. Beet and Goat Cheese Salad

Ingredients:
- 4 medium beets, roasted, peeled, and sliced
- 4 cups mixed greens
- 1/2 cup goat cheese, crumbled
- 1/4 cup walnuts, toasted and chopped
- 2 tablespoons balsamic vinegar
- 1 tablespoon olive oil
- Salt and pepper to taste

Instructions:
1. Arrange the mixed greens on a serving platter or in a salad bowl.
2. Top with sliced beets, crumbled goat cheese, and toasted walnuts.
3. Drizzle with balsamic vinegar and olive oil.
4. Season with salt and pepper to taste and serve immediately.

Serves:
- 4 servings

Nutritional Info (per serving):
- Calories: 250
- Protein: 8g
- Carbohydrates: 13g
- Fat: 18g
- Fiber: 3g
- Calcium: 60mg

Cooking Time:
- Prep Time: 15 minutes (additional time for roasting beets)

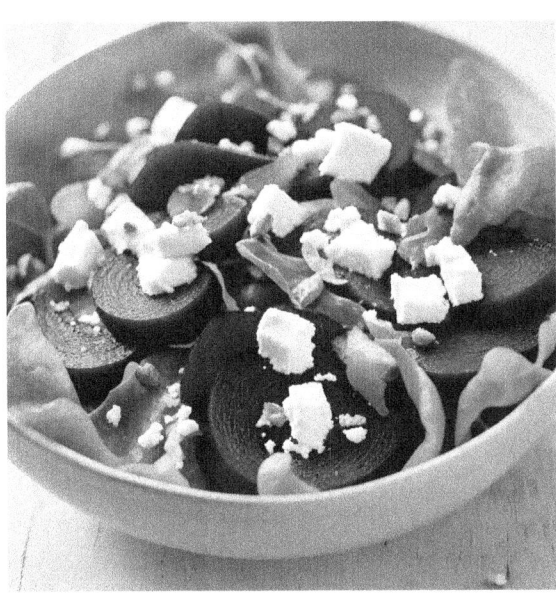

14. Rice and Bean Bowl

Ingredients:
- 2 cups cooked brown rice
- 1 can (15 oz) black beans, rinsed and drained
- 1 cup corn kernels (fresh, frozen, or canned)
- 1 red bell pepper, diced
- 1 avocado, diced
- 1/2 cup fresh cilantro, chopped
- Juice of 1 lime
- 2 tablespoons olive oil
- Salt and pepper to taste

Instructions:
1. Divide the cooked brown rice among 4 bowls.
2. Top each bowl evenly with black beans, corn, diced red bell pepper, and diced avocado.
3. Drizzle with lime juice and olive oil.
4. Garnish with fresh cilantro, and season with salt and pepper to taste.
5. Serve immediately, mixing everything together just before eating.

Serves:
- 4 servings

Nutritional Info (per serving):
- Calories: 350
- Protein: 10g
- Carbohydrates: 55g
- Fat: 11g
- Fiber: 13g
- Calcium: 50mg

Cooking Time:
- Prep Time: 10 minutes (additional time if cooking rice from scratch)

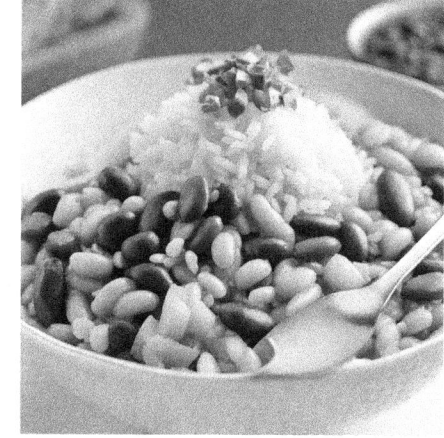

15. Tuna Salad

Ingredients:
- 2 cans (5 oz each) tuna in water, drained
- 1/4 cup mayonnaise (low-fat or avocado-based)
- 1 celery stalk, diced
- 1/4 red onion, finely chopped
- 1 tablespoon lemon juice
- Salt and pepper to taste
- Lettuce leaves for serving

Instructions:
1. In a bowl, mix the drained tuna, mayonnaise, diced celery, and chopped red onion.
2. Add the lemon juice, and season with salt and pepper to taste.
3. Serve the tuna salad on a bed of lettuce leaves or as a sandwich filling.

Serves:
- 4 servings

Nutritional Info (per serving):
- Calories: 180
- Protein: 25g
- Carbohydrates: 2g
- Fat: 8g
- Fiber: 0.5g
- Calcium: 20mg

Cooking Time:
- Prep Time: 10 minutes

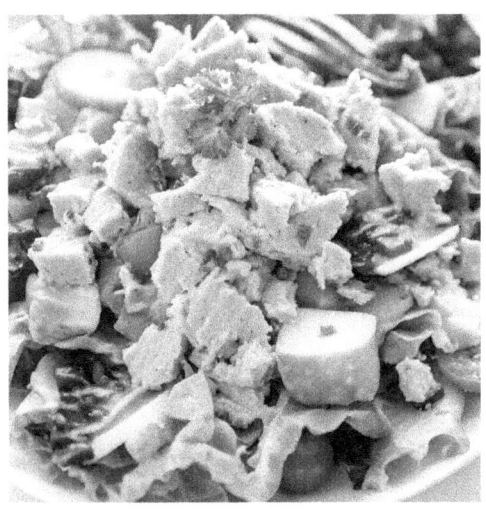

16. Caprese Salad

Ingredients:
- 4 large ripe tomatoes, sliced
- 1 ball fresh mozzarella cheese, sliced
- Fresh basil leaves
- 2 tablespoons balsamic glaze
- 2 tablespoons olive oil
- Salt and pepper to taste

Instructions:
1. Arrange the tomato and mozzarella slices alternately on a platter, overlapping them slightly.
2. Tuck fresh basil leaves between the slices.
3. Drizzle with balsamic glaze and olive oil.
4. Season with salt and pepper just before serving.

Serves:
- 4 servings

Nutritional Info (per serving):
- Calories: 250
- Protein: 10g
- Carbohydrates: 6g
- Fat: 20g
- Fiber: 1g
- Calcium: 200mg

Cooking Time:
- Prep Time: 10 minutes

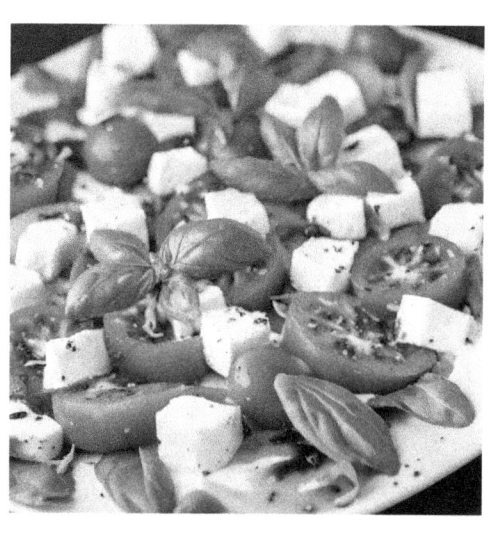

17. Grilled Veggie Sandwich

Ingredients:
- 1 zucchini, sliced lengthwise
- 1 bell pepper, cut into wide strips
- 1 eggplant, sliced into rounds
- 2 tablespoons olive oil
- Salt and pepper to taste
- 4 whole-grain sandwich rolls
- 1/4 cup hummus
- Arugula or lettuce leaves

Instructions:
1. Preheat the grill to medium-high heat.
2. Brush the zucchini, bell pepper, and eggplant slices with olive oil and season with salt and pepper.
3. Grill the vegetables until tender and charred, about 3-4 minutes per side.
4. Spread hummus on the sandwich rolls.
5. Assemble the sandwiches by layering the grilled vegetables and arugula or lettuce on the rolls.
6. Serve immediately or wrap for a picnic or lunch on the go.

Serves:
- 4 servings

Nutritional Info (per serving):
- Calories: 300
- Protein: 8g
- Carbohydrates: 45g
- Fat: 12g
- Fiber: 10g
- Calcium: 80mg

Cooking Time:
- Prep & Cook Time: 20 minutes

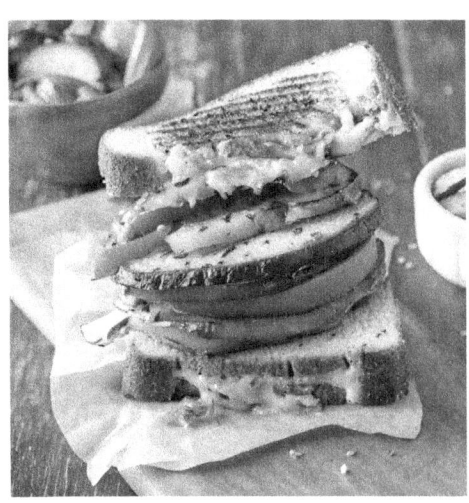

18. Soba Noodle Salad

Ingredients:
- 8 oz soba noodles
- 1 red bell pepper, thinly sliced
- 1 carrot, julienned
- 1 cucumber, julienned
- 3 green onions, chopped
- 1/4 cup soy sauce (or tamari for gluten-free option)
- 2 tablespoons sesame oil
- 1 tablespoon rice vinegar
- 1 tablespoon honey or maple syrup
- 1 teaspoon grated ginger
- Sesame seeds for garnish

Instructions:
1. Cook the soba noodles according to package instructions, then rinse under cold water and drain.
2. In a large bowl, combine the noodles, red bell pepper, carrot, cucumber, and green onions.
3. In a small bowl, whisk together soy sauce, sesame oil, rice vinegar, honey, and ginger to create the dressing.
4. Pour the dressing over the noodle mixture and toss to combine.
5. Sprinkle with sesame seeds before serving.

Serves:
- 4 servings

Nutritional Info (per serving):
- Calories: 320
- Protein: 10g
- Carbohydrates: 56g
- Fat: 8g
- Fiber: 3g
- Calcium: 30mg

Cooking Time:
- Prep & Cook Time: 20 minutes

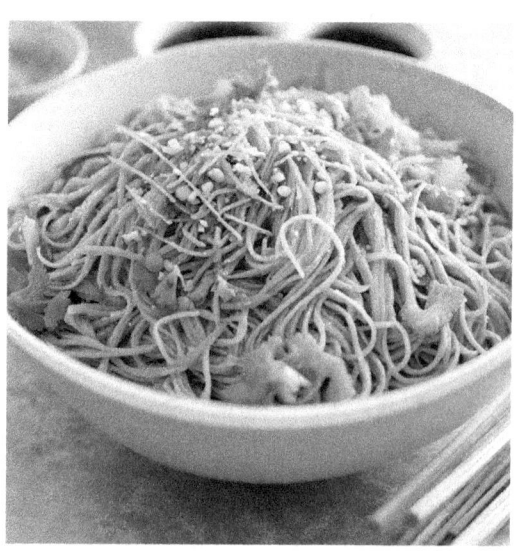

19. Cauliflower Rice Stir-Fry

Ingredients:
- 1 large head cauliflower, grated into "rice"
- 2 tablespoons olive oil
- 1 onion, diced
- 2 garlic cloves, minced
- 1 bell pepper, diced
- 1 cup peas and carrots, frozen or fresh
- 2 eggs, beaten (optional)
- 2 tablespoons soy sauce or tamari
- Salt and pepper to taste
- Green onions and sesame seeds for garnish

Instructions:
1. Heat olive oil in a large skillet over medium heat.
2. Add onion, garlic, and bell pepper. Sauté until softened.
3. Increase heat to medium-high and add the cauliflower rice. Stir-fry for 5-7 minutes.
4. Push the cauliflower mixture to the sides of the skillet, and pour the beaten eggs into the center (if using). Scramble the eggs, then mix into the cauliflower rice.
5. Stir in the peas and carrots, and cook until they are heated through.
6. Add soy sauce, salt, and pepper, adjusting the seasoning to taste.
7. Garnish with green onions and sesame seeds before serving.

Serves:
- 4 servings

Nutritional Info (per serving):
- Calories: 200
- Protein: 8g
- Carbohydrates: 18g
- Fat: 12g
- Fiber: 5g
- Calcium: 60mg

Cooking Time:
- Prep & Cook Time: 25 minutes

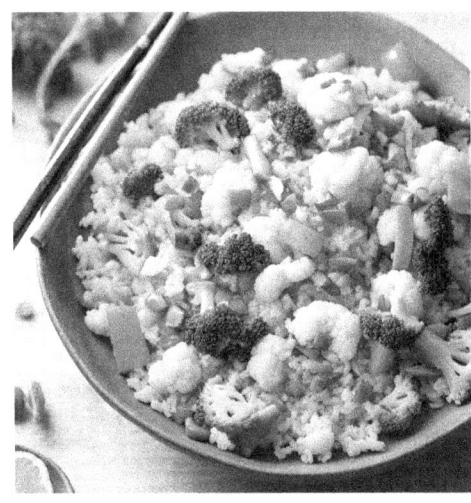

20. Kale and Quinoa Salad

Ingredients:
- 1 cup quinoa, cooked
- 4 cups kale, chopped and massaged
- 1/2 cup cherry tomatoes, halved
- 1/2 cup cucumber, diced
- 1/4 cup red onion, thinly sliced
- 1/4 cup feta cheese, crumbled
- 1/4 cup almonds, chopped
- 3 tablespoons olive oil
- 1 tablespoon lemon juice
- Salt and pepper to taste

Instructions:
1. In a large bowl, combine the cooked quinoa, kale, cherry tomatoes, cucumber, and red onion.
2. Add the feta cheese and almonds on top.
3. In a small bowl, whisk together the olive oil and lemon juice. Season with salt and pepper.
4. Pour the dressing over the salad and toss until everything is well coated.
5. Adjust seasoning as needed and serve.

Serves:
- 4 servings

Nutritional Info (per serving):
- Calories: 330
- Protein: 10g
- Carbohydrates: 34g
- Fat: 18g
- Fiber: 6g
- Calcium: 150mg

Cooking Time:
- Prep Time: 20 minutes

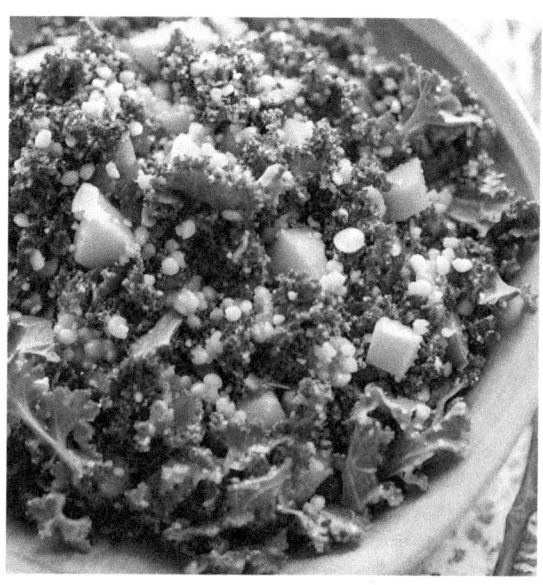

21. Zucchini Noodle Bowl

Ingredients:
- 4 medium zucchinis, spiralized
- 1 tablespoon olive oil
- 1/2 cup cherry tomatoes, halved
- 1/2 cup red bell pepper, sliced
- 1/4 cup olives, sliced
- 1/4 cup feta cheese, crumbled
- 1 tablespoon pesto sauce
- Salt and pepper to taste
- Fresh basil leaves for garnish

Instructions:
1. Heat the olive oil in a large skillet over medium heat
2. Add the spiralized zucchini noodles and sauté for 2-3 minutes until just tender.
3. Stir in the cherry tomatoes, red bell pepper, and olives, cooking for an additional minute.
4. Remove from heat and mix in the pesto sauce, ensuring all the noodles and vegetables are well coated.
5. Season with salt and pepper to taste.
6. Serve the noodles in bowls, topped with crumbled feta cheese and garnished with fresh basil leaves..

Serves:
- 4 servings

Nutritional Info (per serving):
- Calories: 150
- Protein: 4g
- Carbohydrates: 10g
- Fat: 10g
- Fiber: 3g
- Calcium: 100mg

Cooking Time:
- Prep & Cook Time: 15 minutes

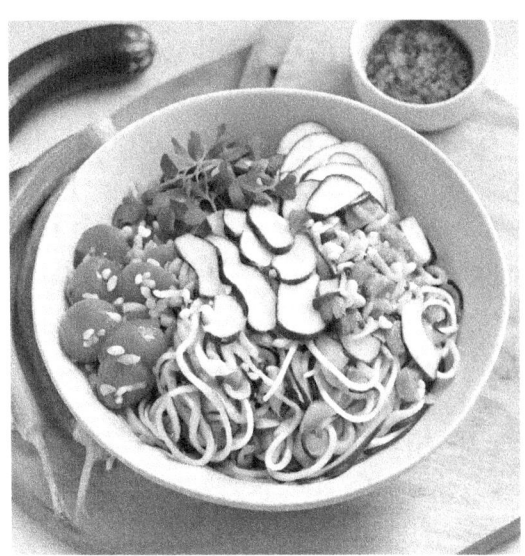

22. Mushroom Risotto

Ingredients:
- 1 cup Arborio rice
- 2 tablespoons olive oil
- 1 onion, finely chopped
- 2 garlic cloves, minced
- 1 pound mushrooms, sliced
- 4 cups vegetable broth, warmed
- 1/2 cup white wine (optional)
- 1/4 cup grated Parmesan cheese
- Salt and pepper to taste
- Fresh parsley, chopped for garnish

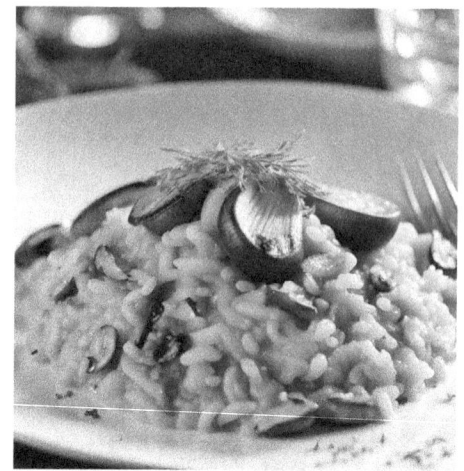

Instructions:
1. Heat 1 tablespoon of olive oil in a large pan over medium heat. Add the onion and garlic, sautéing until soft.
2. Add the mushrooms and cook until they are golden brown. Remove them from the pan and set aside.
3. In the same pan, add another tablespoon of olive oil and the Arborio rice. Stir for 2 minutes until the rice is well-coated and opaque.
4. Pour in the white wine, if using, and let it simmer until the liquid has almost evaporated.
5. Add the warmed vegetable broth, one ladle at a time, stirring continuously, allowing the rice to absorb the liquid before adding more.
6. Once the rice is cooked al dente and the risotto is creamy, stir in the cooked mushrooms, Parmesan cheese, salt, and pepper.
7. Serve hot, garnished with fresh parsley.

Serves:
- 4 servings

Nutritional Info (per serving):
- Calories: 380
- Protein: 12g
- Carbohydrates: 58g
- Fat: 10g
- Fiber: 3g
- Calcium: 80mg

Cooking Time:
- Prep & Cook Time: 45 minutes

23. Spinach and Feta Stuffed Salmon

Ingredients:
- 4 salmon fillets, about 6 oz each
- 2 cups fresh spinach, chopped
- 1/2 cup feta cheese, crumbled
- 2 tablespoons cream cheese, softened
- 1 garlic clove, minced
- Salt and pepper to taste
- 1 tablespoon olive oil

Instructions:
1. Preheat the oven to 375°F (190°C).
2. In a bowl, mix together the spinach, feta cheese, cream cheese, and garlic. Season with salt and pepper.
3. Cut a slit in each salmon fillet to create a pocket. Stuff the pockets evenly with the spinach mixture.
4. Place the stuffed fillets on a baking sheet, drizzle with olive oil, and season with salt and pepper.
5. Bake for 15-20 minutes or until the salmon is cooked through and flakes easily with a fork.
6. Serve immediately, garnished with additional fresh spinach if desired.

Serves:
- 4 servings

Nutritional Info (per serving):
- Calories: 350
- Protein: 35g
- Carbohydrates: 2g
- Fat: 22g
- Fiber: 1g
- Calcium: 100mg

Cooking Time:
- Prep & Cook Time: 30 minutes

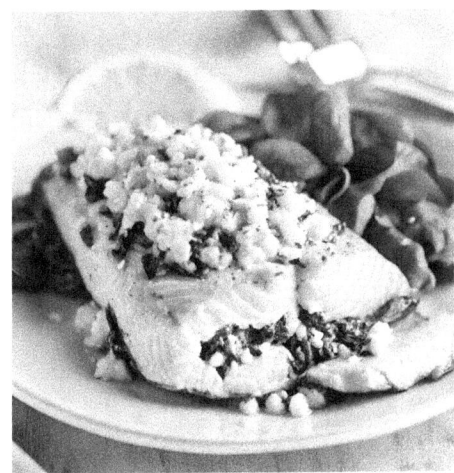

24. Greek Lentil Salad

Ingredients:
- 2 cups cooked lentils
- 1 cucumber, diced
- 1 bell pepper, diced
- 1/2 red onion, finely chopped
- 1 cup cherry tomatoes, halved
- 1/2 cup Kalamata olives, pitted and sliced
- 1/2 cup feta cheese, crumbled
- 1/4 cup olive oil
- 3 tablespoons red wine vinegar
- 1 teaspoon dried oregano
- Salt and pepper to taste
- Fresh parsley, chopped for garnish

Instructions:
1. In a large bowl, combine the cooked lentils, cucumber, bell pepper, red onion, cherry tomatoes, and Kalamata olives.
2. In a small bowl, whisk together the olive oil, red wine vinegar, oregano, salt, and pepper to create the dressing.
3. Pour the dressing over the salad and toss to combine.
4. Gently fold in the crumbled feta cheese.
5. Let the salad sit for at least 10 minutes to allow the flavors to meld, or refrigerate for later serving.
6. Garnish with fresh parsley before serving.

Serves:
- 4 servings

Nutritional Info (per serving):
- Calories: 320
- Protein: 14g
- Carbohydrates: 30g
- Fat: 17g
- Fiber: 12g
- Calcium: 150mg

Cooking Time:
- Prep Time: 15 minutes (plus time to cook lentils if starting from scratch)

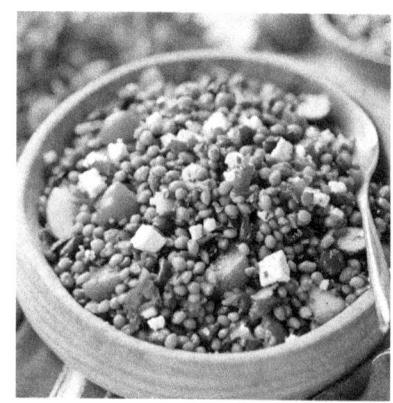

25. Chickpea Vegetable Patties

Ingredients:
- 1 can (15 oz) chickpeas, drained and rinsed
- 1 carrot, grated
- 1 zucchini, grated and excess water squeezed out
- 2 green onions, finely chopped
- 2 garlic cloves, minced
- 1/4 cup fresh parsley, chopped
- 1 teaspoon cumin
- Salt and pepper to taste
- 1 egg, beaten
- 1/2 cup breadcrumbs or oat flour
- 2 tablespoons olive oil for cooking

Instructions:
1. Mash the chickpeas in a large bowl using a fork or potato masher until mostly smooth.
2. Add the grated carrot, zucchini, green onions, garlic, parsley, cumin, salt, and pepper. Mix until well combined.
3. Stir in the beaten egg and breadcrumbs until the mixture holds together. If the mixture is too wet, add more breadcrumbs; if too dry, a little water.
4. Form the mixture into patties, about 3-4 inches in diameter.
5. Heat the olive oil in a large skillet over medium heat. Cook the patties for 3-4 minutes on each side, or until golden brown and heated through.
6. Serve the patties hot, with your choice of sauce or as a burger.

Serves:
- 4 servings (2 patties each)

Nutritional Info (per serving):
- Calories: 290
- Protein: 10g
- Carbohydrates: 35g
- Fat: 13g
- Fiber: 8g
- Calcium: 80mg

Cooking Time:
- Prep & Cook Time: 30 minutes

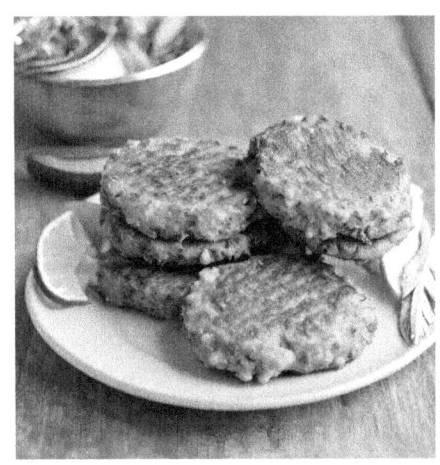

VEGETABLES

1. Roasted Cauliflower Steaks

Ingredients:
- 1 large head cauliflower
- 2 tablespoons olive oil
- Salt and pepper to taste
- 1 teaspoon garlic powder
- 1 teaspoon smoked paprika

Instructions:
1. Preheat the oven to 400°F (200°C).
2. Slice the cauliflower into 1-inch thick steaks, keeping the stem intact to hold the steaks together.
3. Place the cauliflower steaks on a baking sheet. Brush both sides with olive oil and season with salt, pepper, garlic powder, and smoked paprika.
4. Roast for 25-30 minutes, flipping halfway through, until golden brown and tender.

Serves:
- 4 servings

Nutritional Info (per serving):
- Calories: 120
- Protein: 4g
- Carbohydrates: 11g
- Fat: 7g
- Fiber: 5g
- Calcium: 32mg

Cooking Time:
- Prep & Cook Time: 35 minutes

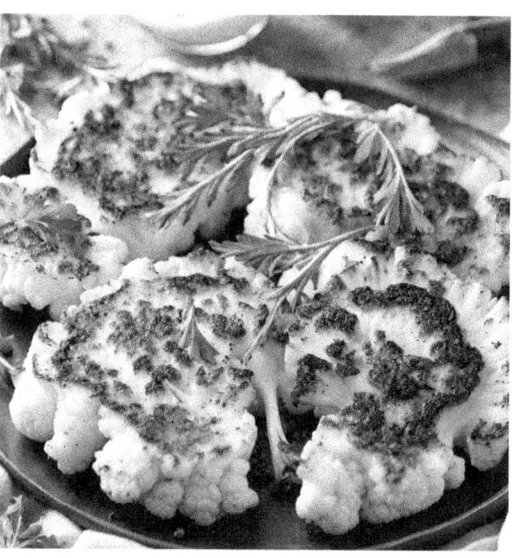

2. Asparagus and Lemon Risotto

Ingredients:
- 1 cup Arborio rice
- 1 bunch asparagus, trimmed and cut into 1-inch pieces
- 4 cups vegetable broth, warmed
- 1 onion, finely chopped
- 2 tablespoons olive oil
- 1/2 cup dry white wine (optional)
- Juice and zest of 1 lemon
- 1/4 cup grated Parmesan cheese
- Salt and pepper to taste

Instructions:
1. In a large skillet, heat the olive oil over medium heat. Add the onion and sauté until translucent.
2. Stir in the Arborio rice, coating it with the oil. Add the white wine and cook until evaporated.
3. Add the warm broth, one ladle at a time, stirring continuously until the liquid is absorbed before adding more.
4. When the rice is halfway cooked, add the asparagus. Continue adding broth and stirring until the rice is creamy and al dente.
5. Remove from heat, stir in the lemon juice, zest, and Parmesan cheese. Season with salt and pepper.
6. Serve immediately, garnished with additional lemon zest if desired.

Serves:
- 4 servings

Nutritional Info (per serving):
- Calories: 320
- Protein: 9g
- Carbohydrates: 53g
- Fat: 7g
- Fiber: 3g
- Calcium: 80mg

Cooking Time:
- Prep & Cook Time: 45 minutes

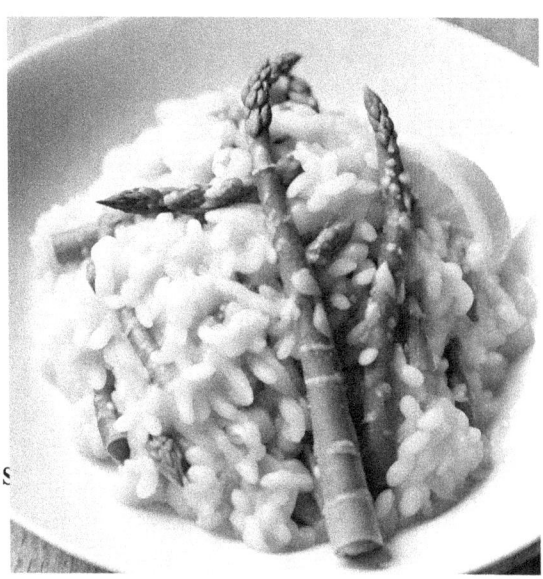

3. Brussels Sprouts with Balsamic Glaze

Ingredients:
- 1 lb Brussels sprouts, halved
- 2 tablespoons olive oil
- Salt and pepper to taste
- 1/4 cup balsamic vinegar
- 2 tablespoons honey or maple syrup

Instructions:
1. Preheat the oven to 400°F (200°C).
2. Toss the Brussels sprouts with olive oil, salt, and pepper. Spread them out on a baking sheet, cut side down.
3. Roast for 20-25 minutes until caramelized and tender.
4. While the Brussels sprouts are roasting, simmer the balsamic vinegar and honey in a small saucepan over low heat until reduced and thickened.
5. Drizzle the glaze over the roasted Brussels sprouts before serving.

Serves:
- 4 servings

Nutritional Info (per serving):
- Calories: 160
- Protein: 4g
- Carbohydrates: 20g
- Fat: 7g
- Fiber: 4g
- Calcium: 48mg

Cooking Time:
- Prep & Cook Time: 30 minutes

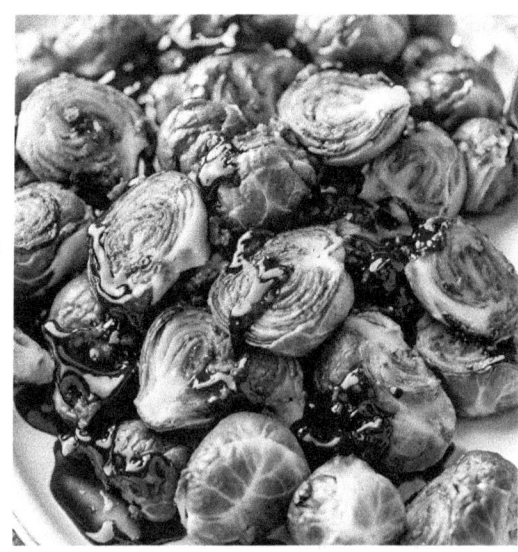

4. Stuffed Acorn Squash

Ingredients:
- 2 acorn squashes, halved and seeded
- 1 tablespoon olive oil
- Salt and pepper to taste
- 1 cup quinoa, cooked
- 1/2 cup cranberries
- 1/2 cup chopped walnuts
- 2 tablespoons maple syrup
- 1 teaspoon cinnamon

Instructions:
1. Preheat the oven to 375°F (190°C). Brush the acorn squash halves with olive oil and season with salt and pepper.
2. Place the squash cut-side down on a baking sheet and roast for 25-30 minutes until tender.
3. Combine the cooked quinoa, cranberries, walnuts, maple syrup, and cinnamon in a bowl.
4. Fill the roasted acorn squash halves with the quinoa mixture.
5. Return the stuffed squashes to the oven and bake for an additional 10 minutes.

Serves:
- 4 servings

Nutritional Info

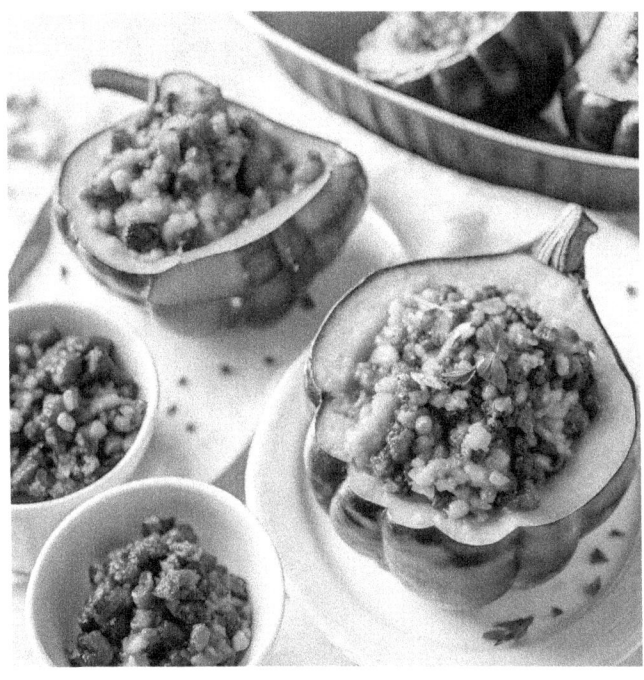

5. Green Beans Almondine

Ingredients:
- 1 lb green beans, trimmed
- 2 tablespoons olive oil
- 1/3 cup sliced almonds
- 2 garlic cloves, minced
- Salt and pepper to taste
- Juice of 1 lemon

Instructions:
1. Blanch the green beans in boiling water for 2-3 minutes until bright green and tender-crisp. Drain and plunge into ice water to stop the cooking process.
2. Heat the olive oil in a large skillet over medium heat. Add the almonds and garlic, sautéing until the almonds are golden and fragrant.
3. Add the drained green beans to the skillet, tossing to coat with the almond and garlic mixture. Cook for an additional 2-3 minutes.
4. Season with salt, pepper, and lemon juice. Toss well and serve immediately.

Serves:
- 4 servings

Nutritional Info (per serving):
- Calories: 160
- Protein: 4g
- Carbohydrates: 10g
- Fat: 12g
- Fiber: 4g
- Calcium: 60mg

Cooking Time:
- Prep & Cook Time: 20 minutes

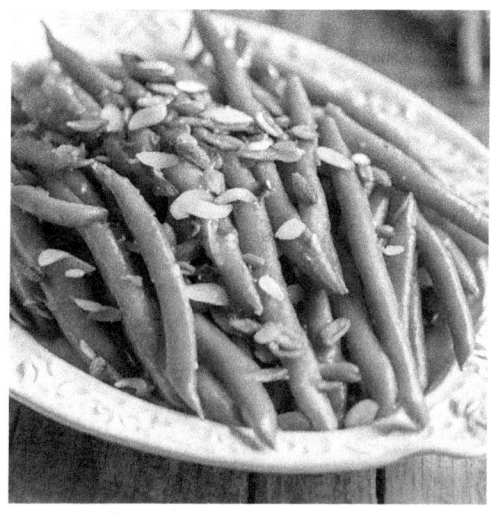

6. Cucumber Tomato Salad

Ingredients:
- 2 large cucumbers, diced
- 3 ripe tomatoes, diced
- 1/4 red onion, thinly sliced
- 1/4 cup olive oil
- 2 tablespoons white wine vinegar
- Salt and pepper to taste
- Fresh herbs (such as parsley or dill), chopped

Instructions:
1. In a large salad bowl, combine the diced cucumbers, tomatoes, and red onion.
2. Whisk together the olive oil and white wine vinegar. Pour over the salad and gently toss to coat.
3. Season with salt, pepper, and fresh herbs. Toss again and adjust seasoning as needed.
4. Chill in the refrigerator for 15-20 minutes before serving to allow flavors to meld.

Serves:
- 4 servings

Nutritional Info (per serving):
- Calories: 140
- Protein: 2g
- Carbohydrates: 8g
- Fat: 12g
- Fiber: 2g
- Calcium: 30mg

Cooking Time:
- Prep Time: 10 minutes (plus chilling time)

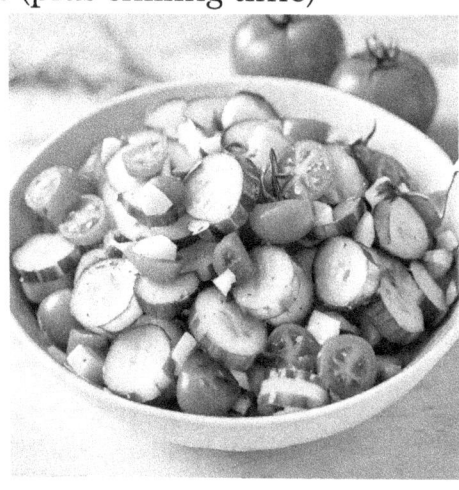

7. Balsamic Roasted Carrots

Ingredients:
- 1 lb carrots, peeled and sliced diagonally
- 2 tablespoons olive oil
- Salt and pepper to taste
- 3 tablespoons balsamic vinegar
- 1 tablespoon honey or maple syrup

Instructions:
1. Preheat the oven to 400°F (200°C).
2. Toss the carrots with olive oil, salt, and pepper, and spread them out on a baking sheet.
3. Roast for 20 minutes, turning once until they start to caramelize.
4. Drizzle with balsamic vinegar and honey. Toss to coat and roast for another 5-10 minutes until glazed and tender.
5. Serve warm, garnished with fresh herbs if desired.

Serves:
- 4 servings

Nutritional Info (per serving):
- Calories: 150
- Protein: 1g
- Carbohydrates: 19g
- Fat: 7g
- Fiber: 4g
- Calcium: 42mg

Cooking Time:
- Prep & Cook Time: 35 minutes

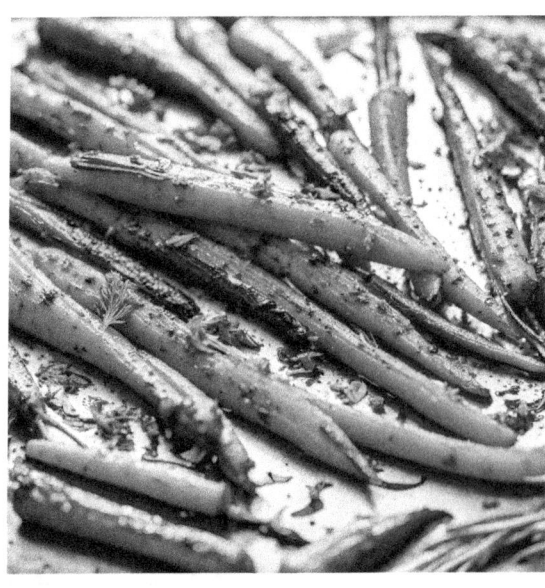

8. Zucchini Boats

Ingredients:
- 4 medium zucchinis, halved lengthwise
- 1 tablespoon olive oil
- 1/2 cup marinara sauce
- 1/2 cup shredded mozzarella cheese (or vegan alternative)
- 1/4 cup grated Parmesan cheese (optional)
- Salt and pepper to taste
- Fresh basil, for garnish

Instructions:
1. Preheat the oven to 375°F (190°C). Scoop out the center of each zucchini half to create a "boat."
2. Brush the zucchini with olive oil and season with salt and pepper. Place them on a baking sheet and bake for 15 minutes until slightly tender.
3. Spoon marinara sauce into each zucchini boat. Sprinkle with mozzarella and Parmesan cheeses.
4. Return to the oven and bake for an additional 10-15 minutes, or until the cheese is melted and bubbly.
5. Garnish with fresh basil before serving.

Serves:
- 4 servings

Nutritional Info(per serving):
- Calories: 180
- Protein: 8g
- Carbohydrates: 10g
- Fat: 12g
- Fiber: 3g
- Calcium: 150mg

Cooking Time:
- Prep & Cook Time: 30 minutes

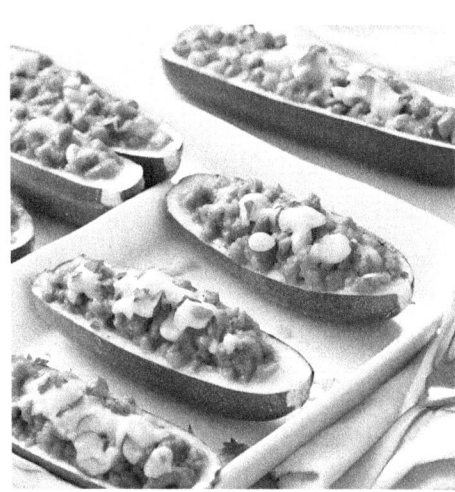

9. Spinach and Mushroom Frittata

Ingredients:
- 8 large eggs
- 2 cups fresh spinach, chopped
- 1 cup mushrooms, sliced
- 1/2 onion, diced
- 1/4 cup milk (or almond milk)
- 1/2 cup grated Parmesan cheese
- 2 tablespoons olive oil
- Salt and pepper to taste

Instructions:
1. Preheat the oven to 375°F (190°C).
2. Heat olive oil in a large oven-safe skillet over medium heat. Add the onions and mushrooms, sautéing until softened.
3. Add the spinach and cook until it wilts.
4. In a bowl, whisk together the eggs, milk, Parmesan, salt, and pepper. Pour the egg mixture over the vegetables in the skillet.
5. Cook over medium heat until the edges start to set, about 5 minutes. Transfer the skillet to the oven.
6. Bake until the frittata is set and lightly golden, about 20-25 minutes. Let it cool slightly before slicing and serving.

Serves:
- 6 servings

Nutritional Info (per serving):
- Calories: 220
- Protein: 14g
- Carbohydrates: 3g
- Fat: 17g
- Fiber: 1g
- Calcium: 150mg

Cooking Time:
- Prep & Cook Time: 40 minutes

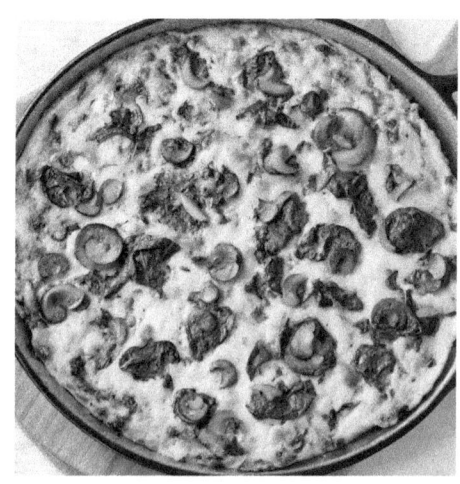

10. Kale Caesar Salad

Ingredients:
- 6 cups kale, stems removed and leaves chopped
- 1/2 cup Caesar dressing (store-bought or homemade, light or vegan version)
- 1/2 cup croutons
- 1/4 cup grated Parmesan cheese (optional)
- Lemon wedges for serving
- Salt and pepper to taste

Instructions:
1. Place the kale in a large bowl. Massage the leaves with your hands for 1-2 minutes to soften.
2. Add the Caesar dressing to the kale and toss to coat evenly. Season with salt and pepper.
3. Top the salad with croutons and Parmesan cheese, if using.
4. Serve with lemon wedges on the side.

Serves:
- 4 servings

Nutritional Info (per serving):
- Calories: 180
- Protein: 6g
- Carbohydrates: 15g
- Fat: 12g
- Fiber: 2g
- Calcium: 130mg

Cooking Time:
- Prep Time: 15 minutes

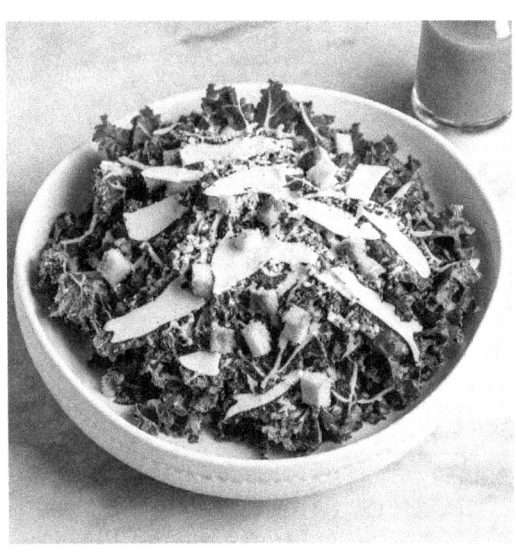

11. Vegetable Paella

Ingredients:
- 2 cups short-grain rice
- 4 cups vegetable broth
- 1 onion, chopped
- 1 red bell pepper, sliced
- 1 yellow bell pepper, sliced
- 1 cup frozen peas
- 1 cup artichoke hearts, quartered
- 3 garlic cloves, minced
- 1 teaspoon saffron threads
- 2 tablespoons olive oil
- Salt and pepper to taste
- Lemon wedges and fresh parsley for garnish

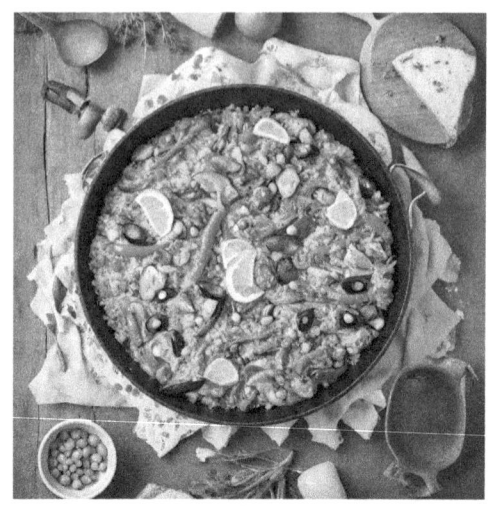

Instructions:
1. Heat the olive oil in a large skillet or paella pan over medium heat. Add the onion, bell peppers, and garlic, sautéing until the vegetables are soft.
2. Add the rice, stirring to coat it with the oil and vegetables. Toast the rice for 2 minutes.
3. Pour in the vegetable broth and sprinkle in the saffron threads. Stir well and bring to a simmer. Reduce the heat to low, cover, and cook for 20 minutes.
4. Add the peas and artichoke hearts, gently folding them into the rice without disturbing the bottom layer. Cook for an additional 10 minutes.
5. Remove from heat and let it sit, covered, for 5-10 minutes. Adjust seasoning with salt and pepper.
6. Serve garnished with lemon wedges and fresh parsley.

Serves:
- 6 servings

Nutritional Info (per serving):
- Calories: 350 Protein: 7g
- Carbohydrates: 65g
- Fat: 7g
- Fiber: 4g
- Calcium: 30mg

Cooking Time:
- Prep & Cook Time: 45 minutes

12. Mushroom Stroganoff

Ingredients:
- 1 lb mushrooms, sliced
- 1 onion, finely chopped
- 2 garlic cloves, minced
- 2 cups vegetable broth
- 1 cup sour cream (or a vegan alternative)
- 2 tablespoons all-purpose flour
- 2 tablespoons olive oil
- 1 tablespoon Worcestershire sauce (vegan if necessary)
- Salt and pepper to taste
- Cooked egg noodles or rice for serving
- Chopped parsley for garnish

Instructions:
1. Heat olive oil in a large skillet over medium heat. Add the onions and garlic, sautéing until they are soft and translucent.
2. Add the mushrooms and cook until they are browned and have released their moisture.
3. Sprinkle the flour over the mushrooms, stirring to combine, and cook for another minute.
4. Gradually stir in the vegetable broth, ensuring there are no lumps. Bring to a simmer, allowing the mixture to thicken slightly.
5. Reduce the heat to low and stir in the sour cream and Worcestershire sauce. Season with salt and pepper, and heat gently until the sauce is hot (do not boil).
6. Serve the stroganoff over cooked egg noodles or rice, garnished with chopped parsley.

Serves:
- 4 servings

Nutritional Info (per serving):
- Calories: 300
- Protein: 6g
- Carbohydrates: 15g
- Fat: 24g
- Fiber: 2g
- Calcium: 80mg

Cooking Time:
- Prep & Cook Time: 30 minutes

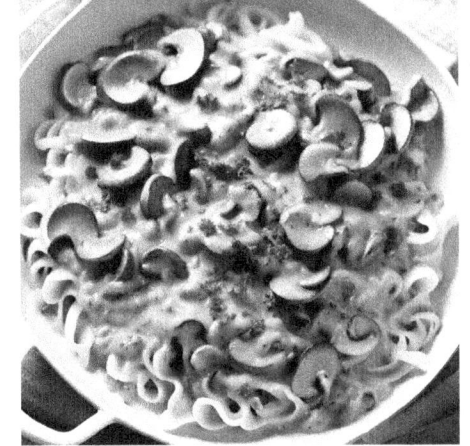

13. Broccoli and Almond Soup

Ingredients:
- 2 tablespoons olive oil
- 1 onion, chopped
- 2 cloves garlic, minced
- 4 cups broccoli florets
- 4 cups vegetable broth
- 1/2 cup almonds, toasted and chopped
- Salt and pepper to taste
- 1/2 cup heavy cream or coconut milk (optional)

Instructions:
1. Heat olive oil in a large pot over medium heat. Add onion and garlic, and sauté until onion is translucent.
2. Add broccoli and cook for 5 minutes, stirring occasionally.
3. Pour in the vegetable broth and bring to a boil. Reduce heat, cover, and simmer for 15-20 minutes, or until broccoli is tender.
4. Use an immersion blender to puree the soup until smooth (or transfer to a blender in batches).
5. Stir in the toasted almonds, and season with salt and pepper. If using, add the cream or coconut milk and heat through.
6. Serve hot, garnished with additional almonds if desired.

Serves:
- 4 servings

Nutritional Info (per serving):
- Calories: 230
- Protein: 6g
- Carbohydrates: 14g
- Fat: 17g
- Fiber: 5g
- Calcium: 70mg

Cooking Time:
- Prep & Cook Time: 40 minutes

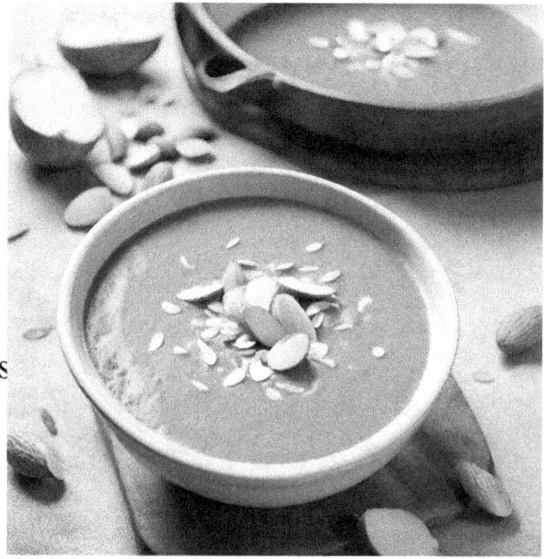

14. Roasted Beet and Walnut Salad

Ingredients:
- 4 medium beets, peeled and diced
- 2 tablespoons olive oil
- Salt and pepper to taste
- 4 cups mixed salad greens
- 1/2 cup walnuts, toasted
- 1/4 cup crumbled goat cheese or feta (optional)
- Balsamic vinaigrette dressing

Instructions:
1. Preheat the oven to 400°F (200°C). Toss the beets with olive oil, salt, and pepper.
2. Spread the beets on a baking sheet and roast for 25-30 minutes, or until tender.
3. Let the beets cool slightly, then combine with the salad greens, walnuts, and goat cheese in a large salad bowl.
4. Drizzle with balsamic vinaigrette, toss to combine, and serve immediately.

Serves:
- 4 servings

Nutritional Info (per serving):
- Calories: 280
- Protein: 7g
- Carbohydrates: 15g
- Fat: 22g
- Fiber: 5g
- Calcium: 60mg

Cooking Time:
- Prep & Cook Time: 40 minutes

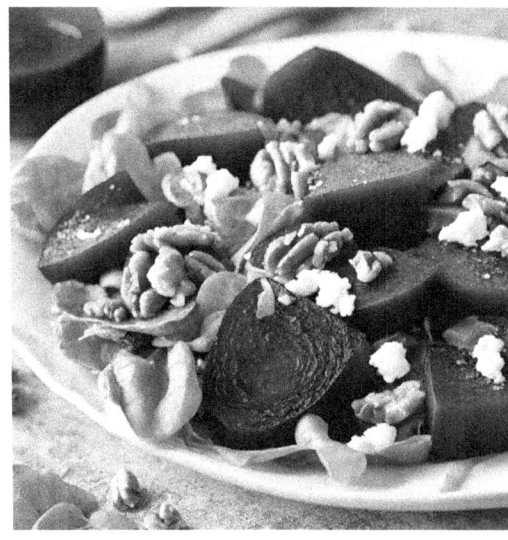

15. Ratatouille

Ingredients:
- 1 eggplant, cubed
- 2 zucchinis, cubed
- 1 bell pepper, chopped
- 1 onion, chopped
- 2 tomatoes, chopped
- 3 cloves garlic, minced
- 1/4 cup olive oil
- 2 teaspoons herbs de Provence or mixed dried herbs
- Salt and pepper to taste
- Fresh basil for garnish

Instructions:
1. Heat olive oil in a large pot or Dutch oven over medium heat. Add the onion and garlic, sautéing until softened.
2. Add the eggplant, zucchini, bell pepper, and tomatoes. Stir in the herbs de Provence, salt, and pepper.
3. Cover and simmer over low heat for 30-40 minutes, stirring occasionally, until vegetables are tender.
4. Adjust seasoning as needed. Serve hot, garnished with fresh basil.

Serves:
- 6 servings

Nutritional Info (per serving):
- Calories: 180
- Protein: 3g
- Carbohydrates: 20g
- Fat: 10g
- Fiber: 6g
- Calcium: 40mg

Cooking Time:
- Prep & Cook Time: 50 minutes

16. Leek and Potato Soup

Ingredients:
- 3 large leeks, cleaned and sliced
- 2 large potatoes, peeled and cubed
- 4 cups vegetable broth
- 2 tablespoons olive oil
- Salt and pepper to taste
- 1 cup light cream or almond milk (optional)
- Chives, chopped (for garnish)

Instructions:
1. Heat the olive oil in a large pot over medium heat. Add the leeks and cook until softened, about 5 minutes.
2. Add the potatoes and vegetable broth. Bring to a boil, then reduce heat and simmer until the potatoes are tender, about 20 minutes.
3. Use an immersion blender to puree the soup until smooth (or use a regular blender, blending in batches).
4. Stir in the light cream or almond milk, if using. Season with salt and pepper.
5. Heat gently, then serve hot, garnished with chives.

Serves:
- 6 servings

Nutritional Info (per serving):
- Calories: 200
- Protein: 3g
- Carbohydrates: 30g
- Fat: 7g
- Fiber: 3g
- Calcium: 50mg

Cooking Time:
- Prep & Cook Time: 35 minutes

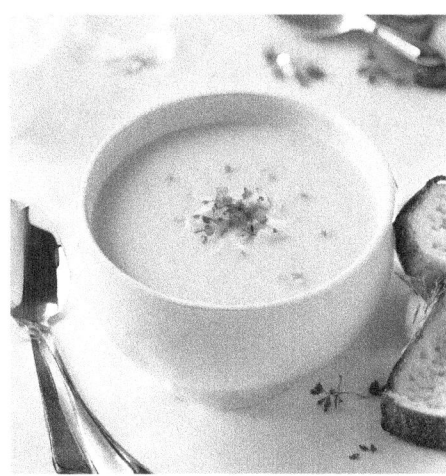

17. Grilled Vegetable Platter

Ingredients:
- 1 zucchini, sliced
- 1 yellow squash, sliced
- 1 red bell pepper, sliced
- 1 eggplant, sliced
- 2 tablespoons olive oil
- Salt and pepper to taste
- Balsamic vinegar or lemon juice (for drizzling)

Instructions:
1. Preheat the grill to medium-high heat.
2. Toss the sliced vegetables with olive oil, salt, and pepper.
3. Grill the vegetables, turning occasionally, until they are tender and have grill marks, about 5-7 minutes per side.
4. Arrange the grilled vegetables on a platter. Drizzle with balsamic vinegar or lemon juice before serving.

Serves:
- 6 servings

Nutritional Info (per serving):
- Calories: 120
- Protein: 2g
- Carbohydrates: 15g
- Fat: 7g
- Fiber: 5g
- Calcium: 30mg

Cooking Time:
- Prep & Cook Time: 20 minutes

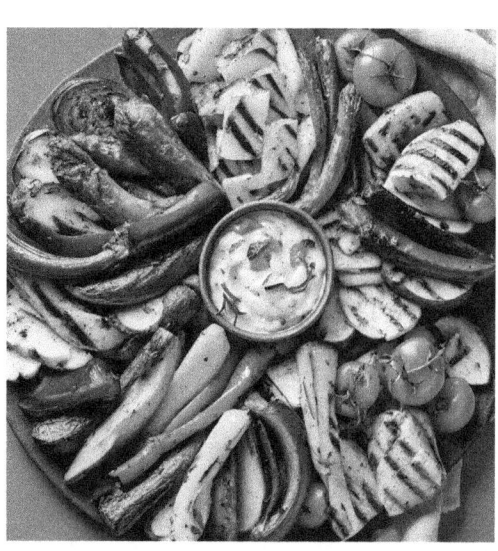

18. Sweet Potato Rounds

Ingredients:
- 2 large sweet potatoes, sliced into rounds
- 2 tablespoons olive oil
- Salt and pepper to taste
- Optional toppings: Greek yogurt, chopped nuts, fresh herbs

Instructions:
1. Preheat the oven to 400°F (200°C).
2. Toss the sweet potato rounds with olive oil, salt, and pepper.
3. Arrange the rounds in a single layer on a baking sheet.
4. Roast for 25-30 minutes, flipping halfway through, until golden and tender.
5. Serve warm with optional toppings like a dollop of Greek yogurt, chopped nuts, or fresh herbs.

Serves:
- 4 servings

Nutritional Info (per serving):
- Calories: 180
- Protein: 2g
- Carbohydrates: 27g
- Fat: 7g
- Fiber: 4g
- Calcium: 40mg

Cooking Time:
- Prep & Cook Time: 35 minutes

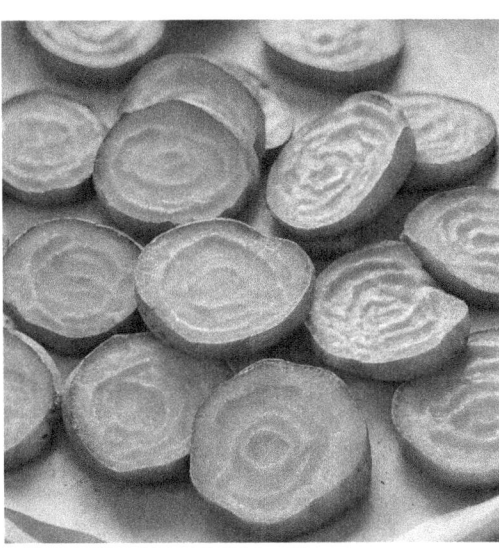

19. Collard Greens with Garlic

Ingredients:
- 1 bunch collard greens, stems removed and leaves chopped
- 3 cloves garlic, minced
- 2 tablespoons olive oil
- Salt and pepper to taste
- 1 tablespoon apple cider vinegar

Instructions:
1. Heat the olive oil in a large skillet over medium heat. Add the garlic and sauté until fragrant, about 1 minute.
2. Add the collard greens and cook, stirring occasionally, until they are wilted and tender, about 10-15 minutes.
3. Season with salt, pepper, and apple cider vinegar. Stir well and cook for another 2 minutes.
4. Serve hot as a nutritious side dish.

Serves:
- 4 servings

Nutritional Info (per serving):
- Calories: 110
- Protein: 3g
- Carbohydrates: 7g
- Fat: 9g
- Fiber: 4g
- Calcium: 150mg

Cooking Time:
- Prep & Cook Time: 20 minutes

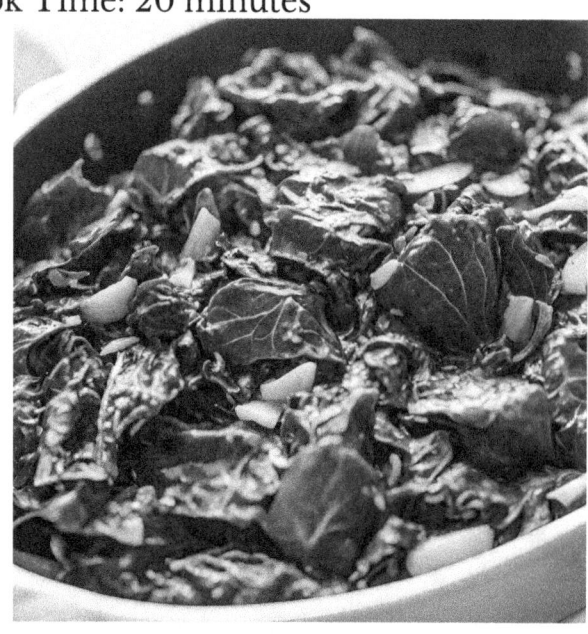

20. Artichoke and Spinach Dip

Ingredients:
- 1 can (14 oz) artichoke hearts, drained and chopped
- 2 cups fresh spinach, chopped
- 1 cup sour cream (or vegan alternative)
- 1 cup cream cheese (or vegan alternative), softened
- 1/2 cup grated Parmesan cheese (optional)
- 2 cloves garlic, minced
- Salt and pepper to taste
- 1 tablespoon olive oil

Instructions:
1. Preheat the oven to 375°F (190°C).
2. In a skillet, heat olive oil over medium heat. Add garlic and sauté until fragrant, about 1 minute.
3. Add spinach and cook until wilted, about 3-5 minutes. Remove from heat.
4. In a mixing bowl, combine the artichoke hearts, sautéed spinach, sour cream, cream cheese, and Parmesan cheese. Season with salt and pepper, and mix until well combined.
5. Transfer the mixture to a baking dish and smooth the top with a spatula.
6. Bake for 20-25 minutes, or until the top is lightly golden and the dip is bubbly.
7. Serve warm with vegetable sticks, whole-grain crackers, or toasted bread.

Serves:
- 8 servings

Nutritional Info (per serving):
- Calories: 220
- Protein: 6g
- Carbohydrates: 7g
- Fat: 19g
- Fiber: 1g
- Calcium: 120mg

Cooking Time:
- Prep & Cook Time: 35 minutes

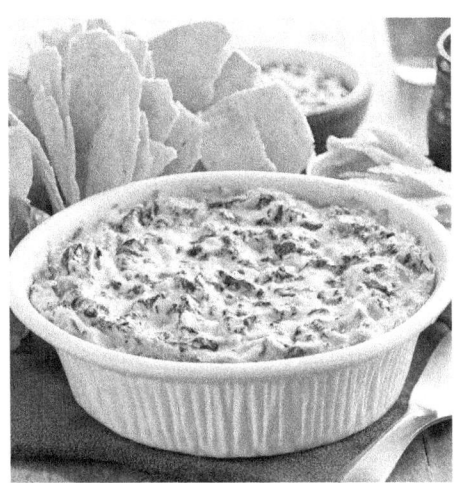

21. Roasted Parsnips with Rosemary

Ingredients:
- 1 lb parsnips, peeled and sliced into batons
- 2 tablespoons olive oil
- 2 teaspoons fresh rosemary, chopped
- Salt and pepper to taste

Instructions:
1. Preheat the oven to 425°F (220°C).
2. In a large bowl, toss the parsnips with olive oil, rosemary, salt, and pepper until well coated.
3. Spread the parsnips out in a single layer on a baking sheet.
4. Roast for 25-30 minutes, turning once halfway through, until golden brown and tender.
5. Serve hot, seasoned with additional salt and pepper if desired.

Serves:
- 4 servings

Nutritional Info (per serving):
- Calories: 140
- Protein: 1g
- Carbohydrates: 20g
- Fat: 7g
- Fiber: 6g
- Calcium: 36mg

Cooking Time:
- **Prep & Cook Time**: 40 minutes

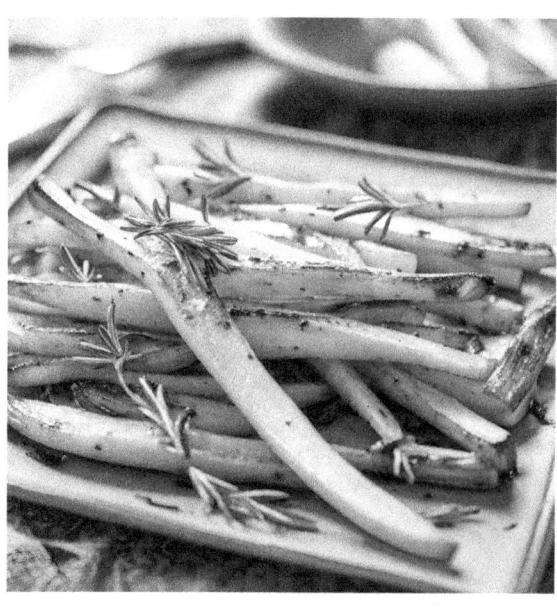

Desserts

1. Baked Apples

Ingredients:
- 4 large apples, cored
- 1/4 cup brown sugar
- 1 teaspoon cinnamon
- 1/4 cup chopped walnuts or pecans (optional)
- 1/4 cup raisins (optional)
- 1 cup apple juice or water

Instructions:
1. Preheat the oven to 350°F (175°C).
2. Mix the brown sugar, cinnamon, walnuts, and raisins in a small bowl.
3. Place the apples in a baking dish and stuff each apple with the sugar mixture.
4. Pour the apple juice or water into the bottom of the dish.
5. Bake for 30-40 minutes, or until the apples are tender but not mushy.
6. Serve warm, spooning the liquid from the baking dish over the apples.

Serves:
- 4 servings

Nutritional Info (per serving):
- Calories: 200
- Protein: 1g
- Carbohydrates: 50g
- Fat: 2g (if using nuts)
- Fiber: 5g
- Calcium: 20mg

Cooking Time:
- Prep & Cook Time: 45 minutes

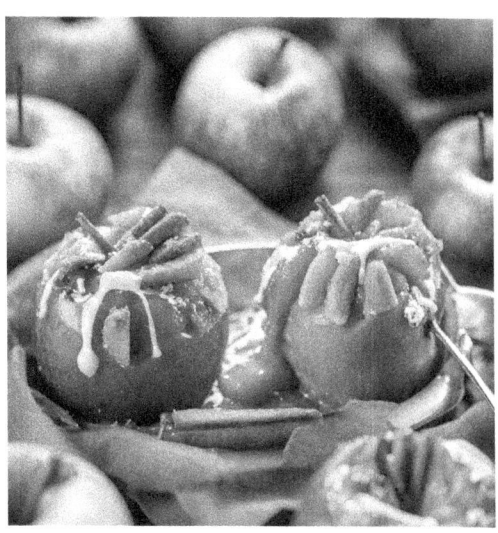

2. Pineapple Sorbet

Ingredients:
- 1 large pineapple, peeled, cored, and chopped
- 1/4 cup sugar (adjust according to taste)
- 1 tablespoon lime juice

Instructions:
1. Blend the pineapple chunks in a food processor or blender until smooth.
2. Mix in the sugar and lime juice, and blend again.
3. Pour the mixture into an ice cream maker and churn according to the manufacturer's instructions. If you don't have an ice cream maker, freeze the mixture for 1-2 hours, then blend again to break up ice crystals. Repeat the freeze and blend process 2-3 times.
4. Once the sorbet is smooth and frozen, transfer it to a freezer-safe container and freeze until firm.
5. Let it sit at room temperature for a few minutes before serving to soften slightly.

Serves:
- 6 servings

Nutritional Info (per serving):
- Calories: 120
- Protein: 1g
- Carbohydrates: 30g
- Fat: 0g
- Fiber: 2g
- Calcium: 20mg

Cooking Time:
- Prep & Freeze Time: Varies depending on the method, approximately 2-4 hours

3. Rice Pudding

Ingredients:
- 1/2 cup uncooked white rice
- 4 cups milk (or almond milk for a dairy-free version)
- 1/3 cup sugar
- 1/4 teaspoon salt
- 1/2 teaspoon vanilla extract
- Cinnamon or nutmeg for garnish (optional)

Instructions:
1. In a saucepan, combine the rice, milk, sugar, and salt.
2. Bring to a boil over medium heat, then reduce to a simmer, stirring frequently to prevent the rice from sticking.
3. Cook until the rice is tender and the mixture has thickened, about 25-30 minutes.
4. Remove from heat and stir in the vanilla extract.
5. Pour into serving dishes and sprinkle with cinnamon or nutmeg if desired.
6. Serve warm or chill in the refrigerator before serving.

Serves:
- 6 servings

Nutritional Info (per serving):
- Calories: 200
- Protein: 5g
- Carbohydrates: 35g
- Fat: 4g (using almond milk)
- Fiber: 0g
- Calcium: 150mg (using almond milk)

Cooking Time:
- Prep & Cook Time: 40 minutes

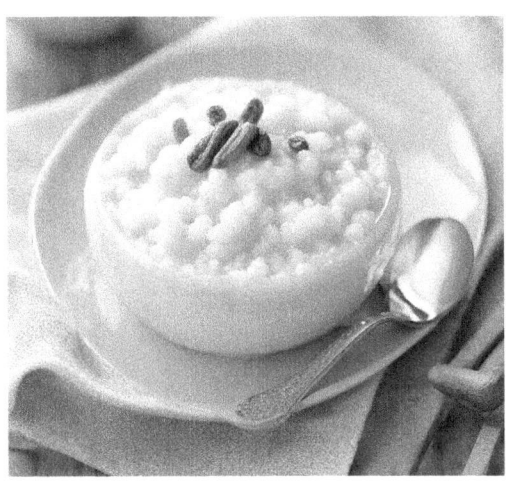

4. Poached Pears

Ingredients:
- 4 firm pears, peeled, halved, and cored
- 4 cups water
- 1 cup sugar
- 2 tablespoons lemon juice
- 1 cinnamon stick
- Vanilla extract or vanilla bean (optional)

Instructions:
1. In a large saucepan, combine water, sugar, lemon juice, cinnamon stick, and vanilla.
2. Bring to a simmer over medium heat, stirring until the sugar dissolves.
3. Add the pear halves and simmer gently for 15-20 minutes, or until the pears are tender.
4. Remove the pears and reduce the liquid to create a syrup.
5. Serve the pears drizzled with the reduced syrup.

Serves:
- 8 servings (half a pear per serving)

Nutritional Info (per serving):
- Calories: 150
- Protein: 0g
- Carbohydrates: 40g
- Fat: 0g
- Fiber: 3g
- Calcium: 20mg

Cooking Time:
Prep & Cook Time: 30 minutes

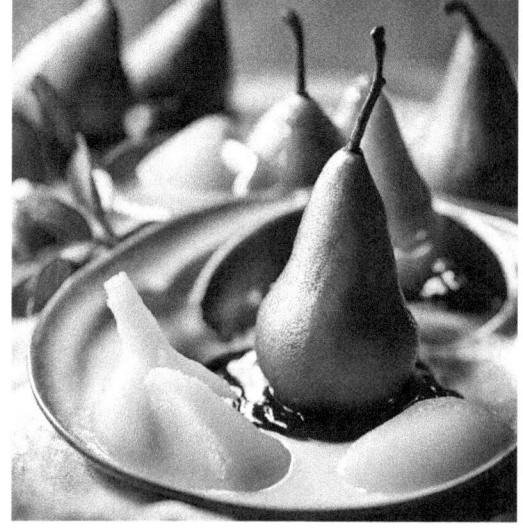

5. Angel Food Cake

Ingredients:
- 1 cup cake flour
- 1 1/2 cups granulated sugar, divided
- 12 large egg whites, room temperature
- 1 1/2 teaspoons cream of tartar
- 1/4 teaspoon salt
- 1 teaspoon vanilla extract

Instructions:
1. Preheat the oven to 350°F (175°C).
2. Sift the cake flour and 3/4 cup of sugar together twice and set aside.
3. In a large bowl, beat the egg whites with the cream of tartar and salt until foamy.
4. Gradually add the remaining 3/4 cup of sugar, continuing to beat until stiff peaks form.
5. Fold in the vanilla extract.
6. Gradually sift the flour-sugar mixture over the egg whites and gently fold it in, being careful not to deflate the mixture.
7. Spoon the batter into an ungreased 10-inch tube pan.
8. Bake for 35-40 minutes, or until the cake springs back when lightly touched.
9. Invert the pan and allow the cake to cool completely before removing it from the pan.
10. Serve as is or with fresh fruit and whipped cream.

Serves:
- 12 servings

Nutritional Info (per serving):
- Calories: 160
- Protein: 4g
- Carbohydrates: 35g
- Fat: 0g
- Fiber: 0g
- Calcium: 5mg

Cooking Time:
- Prep & Cook Time: 1 hour

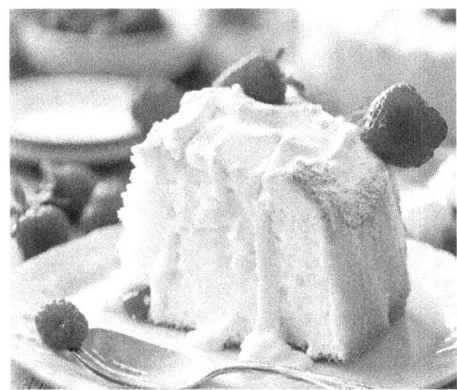

6. Pumpkin Mousse
Ingredients:
- 1 can (15 oz) pure pumpkin puree
- 1 teaspoon pumpkin pie spice
- 1/2 cup granulated sugar
- 1 1/2 cups heavy whipping cream (or a dairy-free alternative)
- 1 teaspoon vanilla extract

Instructions:
1. In a large bowl, mix together the pumpkin puree, pumpkin pie spice, and sugar until well combined.
2. In a separate bowl, whip the heavy cream and vanilla extract until stiff peaks form.
3. Gently fold the whipped cream into the pumpkin mixture until no streaks remain.
4. Spoon the mousse into individual serving dishes and refrigerate for at least 2 hours, or until set.
5. Garnish with a sprinkle of pumpkin pie spice or a dollop of whipped cream before serving.

Serves:
- 6 servings

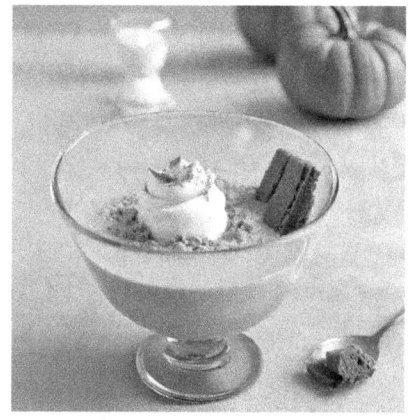

Nutritional Info (per serving):
- Calories: 300
- Protein: 2g
- Carbohydrates: 25g
- Fat: 22g
- Fiber: 2g
- Calcium: 40mg

Cooking Time:
- Prep Time: 15 minutes (plus at least 2 hours chilling)

7. Lemon Jelly

Ingredients:
- 2 cups water
- 1/2 cup lemon juice
- 1/4 cup sugar (adjust to taste)
- 2 1/2 teaspoons agar-agar powder

Instructions:
1. In a saucepan, combine water, lemon juice, and sugar. Heat gently, stirring until the sugar dissolves.
2. Sprinkle the agar-agar powder over the liquid and whisk thoroughly. Bring the mixture to a boil, then simmer for 2 minutes, stirring constantly.
3. Pour the mixture into a mold or individual serving dishes. Allow to cool slightly, then refrigerate until set, about 2 hours.
4. Serve chilled.

Serves:
- 4 servings

Nutritional Info (per serving):
- Calories: 60
- Protein: 0g
- Carbohydrates: 15g
- Fat: 0g
- Fiber: 0g
- Calcium: 5mg

Cooking Time:
- Prep & Chill Time: 2 hours 15 minutes

8. Banana Ice Cream

Ingredients:
- 4 ripe bananas, sliced and frozen

Instructions:
1. Place the frozen banana slices in a food processor or high-powered blender.
2. Pulse until the mixture is smooth and creamy, resembling soft-serve ice cream.
3. Serve immediately for a soft-serve texture or freeze for an additional hour for a firmer consistency.

Serves:
- 4 servings

Nutritional Info (per serving):
- Calories: 105
- Protein: 1g
- Carbohydrates: 27g
- Fat: 0g
- Fiber: 3g
- Calcium: 5mg

Cooking Time:
- Prep Time: 5 minutes (plus freezing time for bananas)

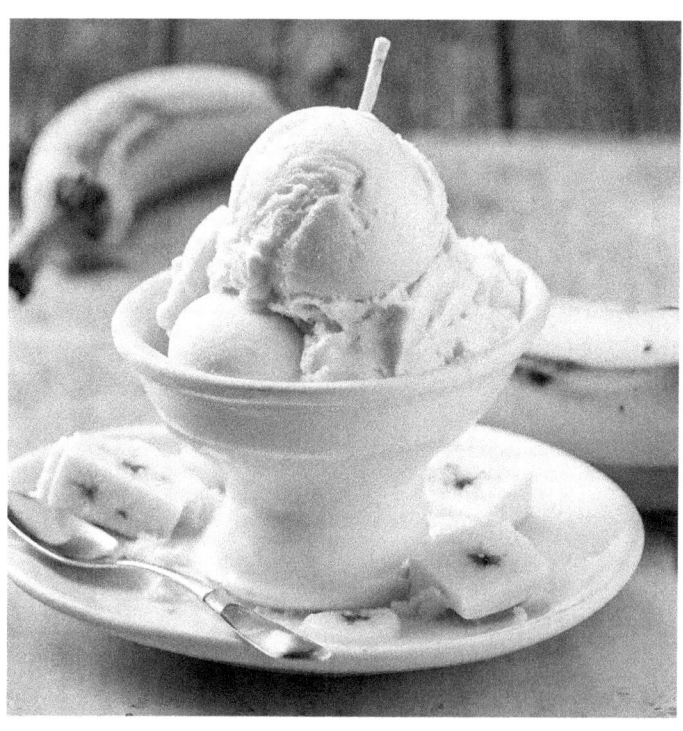

9. Mango Pudding

Ingredients:
- 2 ripe mangoes, peeled and cubed
- 1/2 cup coconut milk
- 1/4 cup sugar
- 2 teaspoons agar-agar powder
- 1/2 cup hot water

Instructions:
1. Dissolve the agar-agar powder in hot water and let it cool slightly.
2. Blend the mangoes, coconut milk, and sugar in a blender until smooth.
3. Mix the mango puree with the agar-agar solution.
4. Pour the mixture into molds or serving dishes and refrigerate until set, about 2-3 hours.
5. Serve chilled.

Serves:
- 4 servings

Nutritional Info (per serving):
- Calories: 150
- Protein: 1g
- Carbohydrates: 28g
- Fat: 5g
- Fiber: 2g
- Calcium: 15mg

Cooking Time:
- Prep & Chill Time: 3 hours

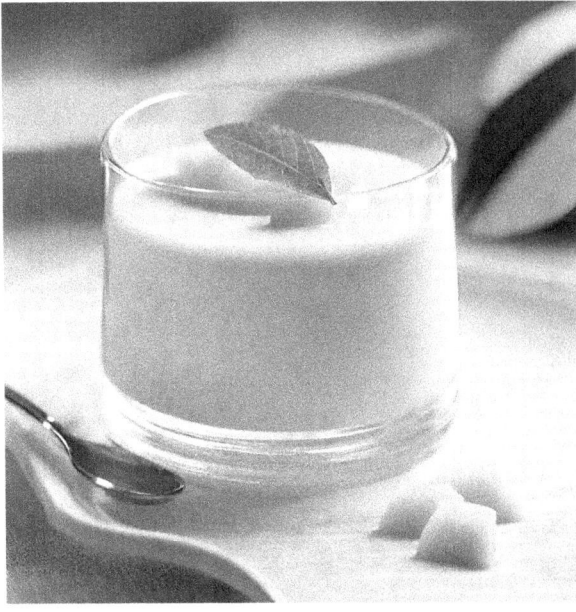

10. Berry Salad

Ingredients:
- 2 cups strawberries, hulled and halved
- 1 cup blueberries
- 1 cup raspberries
- 1 cup blackberries
- 2 tablespoons honey or maple syrup
- 1 tablespoon fresh lemon juice

Instructions:
1. In a large bowl, combine all the berries.
2. Drizzle with honey or maple syrup and lemon juice.
3. Gently toss to combine and coat the berries evenly.
4. Refrigerate for at least 30 minutes before serving to allow the flavors to meld.

Serves:
- 4 servings

Nutritional Info (per serving):
- Calories: 100
- Protein: 1g
- Carbohydrates: 25g
- Fat: 0.5g
- Fiber: 7g
- Calcium: 30mg

Cooking Time:
- Prep Time: 10 minutes (plus chilling time)

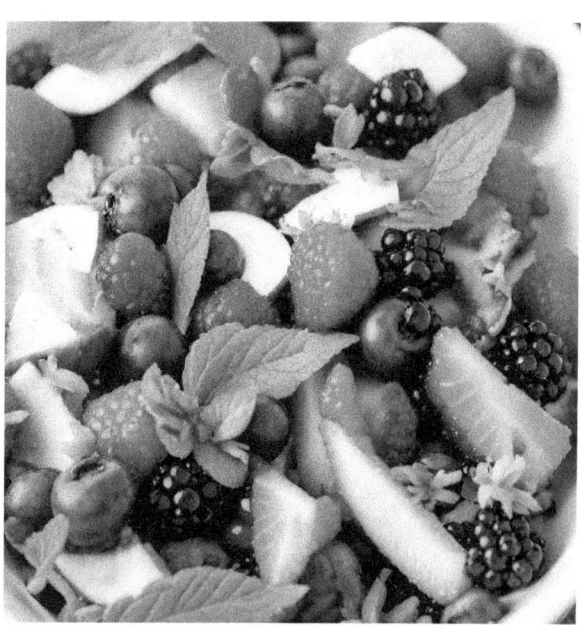

11. Apple Crisp

Ingredients:
- 4 large apples, peeled, cored, and sliced
- 1/2 cup rolled oats
- 1/2 cup flour (whole wheat or almond flour for a healthier option)
- 1/2 cup brown sugar
- 1/2 teaspoon cinnamon
- 1/4 cup unsalted butter, melted

Instructions:
1. Preheat the oven to 350°F (175°C).
2. Arrange apple slices in a baking dish.
3. In a bowl, mix oats, flour, brown sugar, and cinnamon. Stir in melted butter until the mixture resembles coarse crumbs.
4. Sprinkle the oat mixture over the apples.
5. Bake for 30-35 minutes or until the topping is golden brown and the apples are tender.
6. Serve warm, optionally with a scoop of vanilla ice cream.

Serves:
- 6 servings

Nutritional Info (per serving):
- Calories: 250
- Protein: 2g
- Carbohydrates: 45g
- Fat: 8g
- Fiber: 4g
- Calcium: 20mg

Cooking Time:
- Prep & Cook Time: 45 minutes

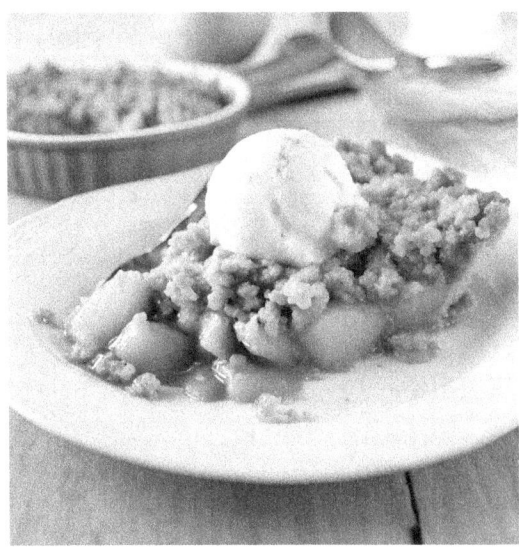

12. Almond Macaroons

Ingredients:
- 1 1/2 cups almond flour
- 1 cup granulated sugar
- 2 large egg whites
- 1/2 teaspoon almond extract
- A pinch of salt

Instructions:
1. Preheat the oven to 325°F (163°C) and line a baking sheet with parchment paper.
2. In a mixing bowl, combine almond flour and sugar.
3. Beat the egg whites with a pinch of salt until stiff peaks form. Fold in the almond extract.
4. Gently fold the egg whites into the almond flour mixture until well combined.
5. Drop spoonfuls of the mixture onto the prepared baking sheet, spacing them about 1 inch apart.
6. Bake for 20-25 minutes, or until the macaroons are golden.
7. Allow to cool on the baking sheet for 5 minutes, then transfer to a wire rack to cool completely.

Serves:
- 15 macaroons

Nutritional Info (per macaroon):
- Calories: 100
- Protein: 3g
- Carbohydrates: 13g
- Fat: 5g
- Fiber: 1g
- Calcium: 20mg

Cooking Time:
- Prep & Cook Time: 30 minutes

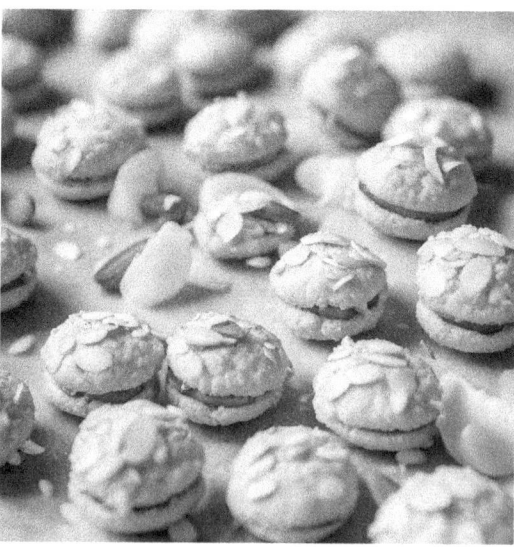

13. Melon Balls

Ingredients:
- 1 cantaloupe
- 1 honeydew melon
- 1 watermelon

Instructions:
1. Using a melon baller, scoop out balls from the cantaloupe, honeydew, and watermelon.
2. Combine the melon balls in a large bowl.
3. Chill in the refrigerator until ready to serve. Optionally, drizzle with a bit of honey or lime juice before serving for added flavor.

Serves:
- 6 servings

Nutritional Info (per serving):
- Calories: 80
- Protein: 1g
- Carbohydrates: 19g
- Fat: 0g
- Fiber: 1g
- Calcium: 20mg

Cooking Time:
- Prep Time: 15 minutes

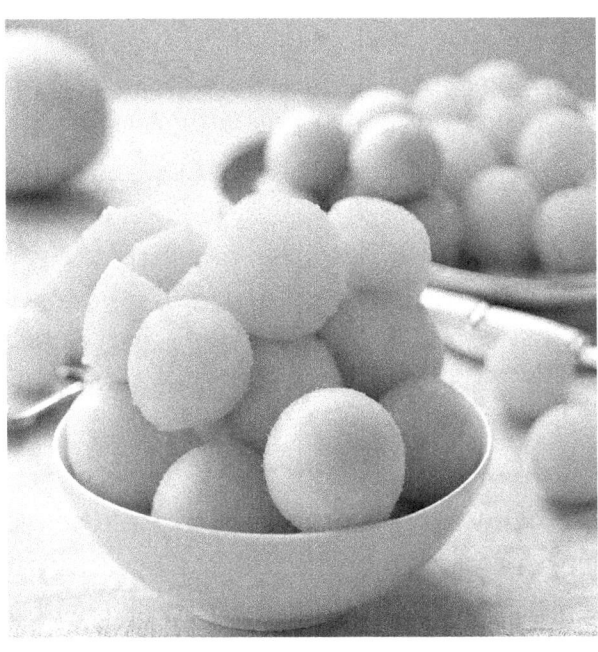

8-WEEK MEAL PLAN

Week 1 Meal Plan

Day 1
- Breakfast: Oatmeal topped with sliced apples and cinnamon; herbal tea.
- Lunch: Quinoa salad with roasted vegetables and feta cheese; pear slices.
- Dinner: Grilled salmon, steamed green beans, and a side salad with lemon vinaigrette.
- Snacks: Carrot sticks and hummus; yogurt.

Day 2
- Breakfast: Greek yogurt with blueberries and a sprinkle of chia seeds.
- Lunch: Turkey and avocado wrap; orange slices.
- Dinner: Baked chicken breast, roasted sweet potatoes, and steamed broccoli.
- Snacks: Sliced cucumbers; apple slices with almond butter.

Day 3
- Breakfast: Scrambled eggs with spinach and mushrooms; whole grain toast.
- Lunch: Lentil soup; side salad with cherry tomatoes and balsamic dressing.
- Dinner: Stir-fried tofu with mixed vegetables over brown rice.
- Snacks: Peach slices; cottage cheese.

Day 4
- Breakfast: Smoothie with banana, kale, and almond milk.
- Lunch: Chicken Caesar salad with a low-fat dressing; kiwi fruit.
- Dinner: Grilled shrimp, quinoa, and asparagus.
- Snacks: Sliced bell peppers; a handful of almonds.

Day 5
- Breakfast: Whole grain pancakes topped with fresh strawberries.
- Lunch: Vegetable lasagna with a side of mixed greens.
- Dinner: Roast turkey, mashed cauliflower, and peas.
- Snacks: Mixed berries; low-fat cheese sticks.

Day 6
- Breakfast: Poached eggs on whole-grain toast; grapefruit slices.
- Lunch: Tuna salad stuffed tomatoes; cucumber salad.
- Dinner: Beef stir-fry with a variety of vegetables over jasmine rice.
- Snacks: Apple slices; yogurt.

Day 7
- Breakfast: Berry and banana smoothie with skim milk.
- Lunch: Mediterranean chickpea salad; watermelon slices.
- Dinner: Baked cod, wild rice, and steamed carrots.
- Snacks: Pear slices; a handful of walnuts.

Week 2 Meal Plan

Day 1
- Breakfast: Chia pudding made with almond milk and topped with raspberries.
- Lunch: Roasted turkey and avocado salad with spinach and a citrus vinaigrette.
- Dinner: Grilled portobello mushrooms, barley salad with cucumbers and tomatoes, and steamed kale.
- Snacks: Kiwi slices; rice cakes with peanut butter.

Day 2
- Breakfast: Breakfast tacos with scrambled eggs, black beans, salsa, and whole grain tortillas.
- Lunch: Soba noodles with stir-fried vegetables and a soy-ginger sauce.
- Dinner: Baked trout with lemon and dill, wild rice, and roasted Brussels sprouts.
- Snacks: Orange slices; a small handful of pumpkin seeds.

Day 3
- Breakfast: Whole grain waffles with a light spread of ricotta cheese and sliced peaches.
- Lunch: Quinoa and black bean stuffed peppers; mixed green salad with vinaigrette.
- Dinner: Lemon-herb roasted chicken, couscous, and steamed green beans.
- Snacks: Banana; a small portion of cottage cheese.

Day 4
- Breakfast: Smoothie bowl with mixed berries, flaxseed, and a swirl of yogurt.
- Lunch: Tuna salad on whole grain bread; carrot and celery sticks.
- Dinner: Vegetarian chili with kidney beans, tomatoes, and corn, served with a side of cornbread.
- Snacks: Apple slices; a few olives.

Day 5
- Breakfast: Poached pear with cinnamon and a dollop of yogurt.
- Lunch: Chicken and vegetable soup; whole grain roll.
- Dinner: Grilled tilapia, quinoa pilaf, and roasted asparagus.
- Snacks: Cucumber slices; a handful of mixed nuts.

Day 6
- Breakfast: Spinach and feta omelet; whole grain toast.
- Lunch: Caprese salad with tomatoes, mozzarella, basil, and balsamic reduction.
- Dinner: Pork tenderloin, baked sweet potato, and sautéed zucchini.
- Snacks: Grapes; a piece of string cheese.

Day 7
- Breakfast: Cottage cheese with sliced pineapple and a sprinkle of toasted coconut.
- Lunch: Roast beef wrap with horseradish cream and arugula; beet salad.
- Dinner: Baked eggplant parmesan, spaghetti squash, and a side salad.
- Snacks: Pear slices; a small serving of almonds.

Week 3 Meal Plan
Day 1
- Breakfast: Avocado toast on whole grain bread with a side of mixed berries.
- Lunch: Lentil and vegetable stew with a slice of rustic bread.
- Dinner: Seared scallops, barley risotto with mushrooms, and roasted butternut squash.
- Snacks: Sliced apples; yogurt with honey.

Day 2
- Breakfast: Quinoa breakfast bowl with sliced almonds and blueberries.
- Lunch: Greek salad with chickpeas, cucumbers, tomatoes, olives, and feta.
- Dinner: Chicken piccata, orzo pasta, and steamed broccoli.
- Snacks: Orange segments; carrot sticks with tzatziki.

Day 3
- Breakfast: Banana and walnut oatmeal with a dash of cinnamon.
- Lunch: Turkey and cranberry sauce sandwich on whole grain bread; kale salad.
- Dinner: Grilled vegetable kebabs, brown rice pilaf, and a side of tzatziki.
- Snacks: Sliced peaches; a small serving of sunflower seeds.

Day 4
- Breakfast: Mixed fruit salad with a dollop of Greek yogurt and a sprinkle of granola.
- Lunch: Roasted chicken breast salad with avocado, bacon, and a hard-boiled egg, dressed lightly.
- Dinner: Pan-seared trout with lemon-caper sauce, farro, and sautéed spinach.
- Snacks: Cucumber slices; a handful of soy nuts.

Day 5
- Breakfast: Spinach, tomato, and goat cheese frittata; whole grain toast.
- Lunch: Asian chicken salad with mandarin oranges, almonds, and a sesame-ginger dressing.
- Dinner: Beef and vegetable stir-fry over quinoa.
- Snacks: Apple slices; a few slices of cheese.

Day 6
- Breakfast: Ricotta and honey spread on whole grain toast with sliced figs.
- Lunch: Shrimp and avocado salad with a lime vinaigrette.
- Dinner: Moroccan spiced chicken, couscous with raisins and carrots, and roasted green beans.
- Snacks: Pear slices; a small serving of pistachios.

Day 7
- Breakfast: Mango and coconut milk smoothie with a scoop of protein powder.
- Lunch: Beet and goat cheese arugula salad with walnuts and a balsamic glaze.
- Dinner: Roasted salmon with a dill yogurt sauce, sweet potato wedges, and steamed peas.
- Snacks: Orange slices; a few slices of cucumber with hummus.

Week 4 Meal Plan
Day 1
- Breakfast: Pear and ginger smoothie with a scoop of vanilla protein powder.
- Lunch: Roasted vegetable and goat cheese frittata; side of mixed greens.
- Dinner: Grilled halibut with a mango salsa, wild rice, and steamed green beans.
- Snacks: Mixed berries; a small serving of cashews.

Day 2
- Breakfast: Scrambled tofu with turmeric, spinach, and tomatoes on whole grain toast.
- Lunch: Chicken gyro salad with tzatziki dressing.
- Dinner: Vegan lentil curry with brown rice and steamed cauliflower.
- Snacks: Carrot sticks; a peach.

Day 3
- Breakfast: Blueberry and almond milk smoothie bowl topped with granola.
- Lunch: Quinoa, black bean, and corn salad with lime vinaigrette.
- Dinner: Turkey meatballs in a tomato sauce with spaghetti squash and a side of asparagus.
- Snacks: Sliced cucumbers; a handful of dried apricots.

Day 4
- Breakfast: Baked sweet potato topped with almond butter and banana slices.
- Lunch: Tabbouleh with fresh parsley, tomatoes, cucumber, and bulgur wheat.
- Dinner: Baked cod with a herb crust, quinoa salad, and roasted Brussels sprouts.

- Snacks: An apple; a few almonds.

Day 5
- Breakfast: Cottage cheese with sliced peaches and a drizzle of honey.
- Lunch: Beef and vegetable stir-fry with brown rice.
- Dinner: Stuffed bell peppers with turkey and vegetables, side of steamed green peas.
- Snacks: Orange slices; a small serving of walnuts.

Day 6
- Breakfast: Avocado and egg breakfast sandwich on whole grain bread.
- Lunch: Mediterranean quinoa bowl with grilled chicken, hummus, and mixed vegetables.
- Dinner: Pork loin roast with apple sauce, mashed potatoes, and steamed carrots.
- Snacks: Kiwi slices; a small serving of sunflower seeds.

Day 7
- Breakfast: Raspberry and flaxseed oatmeal.
- Lunch: Roasted butternut squash soup with a side of whole grain rolls.
- Dinner: Grilled shrimp over a mixed green salad with a lemon-olive oil dressing.
- Snacks: A banana; a small portion of cottage cheese.

Week 5 Meal Plan

Day 1
- Breakfast: Greek yogurt with granola and sliced strawberries.
- Lunch: Avocado tuna salad on mixed greens.
- Dinner: Chicken and vegetable kebabs, brown rice, and a cucumber salad.
- Snacks: Pear slices; a handful of pumpkin seeds.

Day 2
- Breakfast: Smoothie with spinach, pineapple, banana, and coconut water.
- Lunch: Turkey and spinach panini on whole grain bread.
- Dinner: Vegan chickpea stew with sweet potatoes and kale.
- Snacks: Carrot and celery sticks with almond butter.

Day 3
- Breakfast: Egg muffins with bell peppers, onions, and feta cheese.
- Lunch: Asian noodle salad with peanut dressing and shredded chicken.
- Dinner: Baked salmon with a side of farro and steamed broccoli.
- Snacks: An orange; a few slices of cheese.

Day 4
- Breakfast: Chia seed pudding topped with kiwi and coconut flakes.
- Lunch: Grilled chicken Caesar salad with a yogurt-based dressing.
- Dinner: Vegetarian black bean enchiladas with a side of guacamole and salsa.
- Snacks: Sliced apples; a handful of mixed nuts.

Day 5
- Breakfast: Whole grain toast with ricotta, honey, and figs.
- Lunch: Shrimp and avocado wrap with a spicy lime sauce.
- Dinner: Zucchini noodles with turkey meatballs and marinara sauce.
- Snacks: Mixed berries; a small serving of cashews.

Day 6
- Breakfast: Banana nut oatmeal.
- Lunch: Caprese sandwich with tomato, mozzarella, and basil on whole grain bread.
- Dinner: Lemon garlic roasted chicken thighs, couscous, and sautéed green beans.
- Snacks: Grapes; a small serving of almonds.

Day 7
- Breakfast: Pumpkin spice smoothie with almond milk, pumpkin puree, and a scoop of protein powder.
- Lunch: Beef and barley soup with a side salad.
- Dinner: Grilled vegetable platter with hummus and pita bread.
- Snacks: A peach; a few slices of cucumber with hummus.

Week 6 Meal Plan

Day 1
- Breakfast: Overnight oats with almond milk, chia seeds, and mixed berries.
- Lunch: Chicken salad with grapes, walnuts, and celery served on whole grain bread.
- Dinner: Grilled tilapia with lemon butter sauce, quinoa, and steamed spinach.
- Snacks: Carrot sticks; a small serving of cottage cheese.

Day 2
- Breakfast: Multigrain toast with avocado and poached eggs.
- Lunch: Spinach and goat cheese stuffed portobello mushrooms; quinoa tabbouleh.
- Dinner: Slow cooker beef stew with potatoes, carrots, and peas.
- Snacks: An apple; a handful of sunflower seeds.

Day 3
- Breakfast: Protein-packed smoothie with kale, banana, peanut butter, and almond milk.
- Lunch: Mediterranean lentil salad with tomatoes, cucumbers, olives, and feta.
- Dinner: Pan-seared duck breast with orange sauce, wild rice, and roasted parsnips.
- Snacks: Sliced bell peppers; a few olives.

Day 4
- Breakfast: Whole grain pancakes topped with light syrup and fresh blueberries.
- Lunch: Roast beef and horseradish cream on rye with a side of beet salad.
- Dinner: Vegetarian chili served with whole grain cornbread.
- Snacks: A banana; a small portion of almonds.

Day 5
- Breakfast: Greek yogurt with sliced almonds and honey.
- Lunch: Quinoa and roasted vegetable salad with a lemon-tahini dressing.
- Dinner: Turkey lettuce wraps with diced vegetables and hoisin sauce.
- Snacks: Sliced peaches; a small serving of walnuts.

Day 6
- Breakfast: Scrambled eggs with diced tomatoes, onions, and spinach.
- Lunch: Baked sweet potato topped with black beans, salsa, and low-fat sour cream.
- Dinner: Lemon-herb baked cod, barley, and sautéed kale.
- Snacks: Cucumber slices; a handful of pumpkin seeds.

Day 7
- Breakfast: Berry and banana quinoa breakfast bowl.
- Lunch: Grilled vegetable and hummus wrap; side of fruit salad.
- Dinner: Roasted chicken with a side of roasted root vegetables and a mixed green salad.
- Snacks: An orange; a small serving of cashews.

FOOD TRAKER JOURNAL

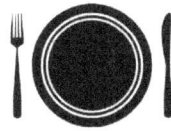

Dates _____

	BREAKFAST	LUNCH	DINNER	SNACKS
MON				
TUE				
WED				
THU				
FRI				
SAT				
SUN				

FOODS TO AVOID

_____
_____
_____
_____
_____

FOODS TO AVOID

_____
_____
_____
_____
_____

SHOPPING LIST

_____
_____
_____
_____
_____

Describe your current eating habits and identify which foods you think might be contributing to your kidney stone risk. How do you feel about modifying these habits?

....

....

....

....

....

....

....

....

....

....

What are your primary goals for adjusting your diet (e.g., reducing kidney stone recurrence, improving overall health)? Write down three specific, measurable objectives you hope to achieve.

....

....

....

....

FOOD TRAKER JOURNAL

Dates _____

	BREAKFAST	LUNCH	DINNER	SNACKS
MON				
TUE				
WED				
THU				
FRI				
SAT				
SUN				

FOODS TO AVOID

_____
_____
_____
_____
_____

FOODS TO AVOID

_____
_____
_____
_____
_____

SHOPPING LIST

_____
_____
_____
_____
_____

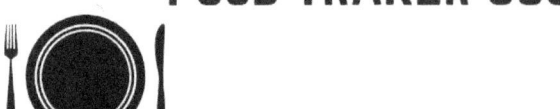
FOOD TRAKER JOURNAL

Dates
_____

	BREAKFAST	LUNCH	DINNER	SNACKS
MON				
TUE				
WED				
THU				
FRI				
SAT				
SUN				

FOODS TO AVOID   FOODS TO AVOID   SHOPPING LIST

_____   _____   _____
_____   _____   _____
_____   _____   _____
_____   _____   _____
_____   _____   _____

List at least five high-oxalate foods you commonly eat. Next to each, brainstorm one or two lower-oxalate alternatives you could try instead.

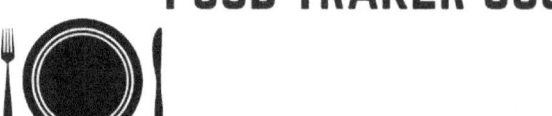
FOOD TRAKER JOURNAL

Dates
_____

	BREAKFAST	LUNCH	DINNER	SNACKS
MON				
TUE				
WED				
THU				
FRI				
SAT				
SUN				

FOODS TO AVOID   **FOODS TO AVOID**   **SHOPPING LIST**

_____   _____   _____
_____   _____   _____
_____   _____   _____
_____   _____   _____
_____   _____   _____

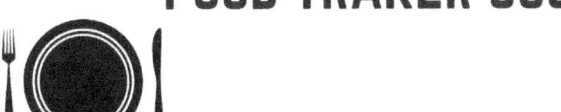
FOOD TRAKER JOURNAL

Dates
_____

	BREAKFAST	LUNCH	DINNER	SNACKS
MON				
TUE				
WED				
THU				
FRI				
SAT				
SUN				

FOODS TO AVOID	FOODS TO AVOID	SHOPPING LIST
_____	_____	_____
_____	_____	_____
_____	_____	_____
_____	_____	_____
_____	_____	_____

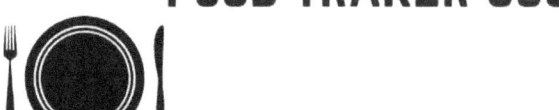

FOOD TRAKER JOURNAL

Dates _____

	BREAKFAST	LUNCH	DINNER	SNACKS
MON				
TUE				
WED				
THU				
FRI				
SAT				
SUN				

FOODS TO AVOID **FOODS TO AVOID** **SHOPPING LIST**

_____   _____   _____
_____   _____   _____
_____   _____   _____
_____   _____   _____
_____   _____   _____

Who in your life can support you in making these dietary changes? Write down ways they can help you stay on track with your kidney stone-friendly diet.

....

....

....

....

....

....

....

....

....

Identify moments when you're most likely to eat for emotional reasons rather than hunger. What healthy coping mechanisms can you develop to address these emotions instead?

....

....

....

....

....

FOOD TRAKER JOURNAL

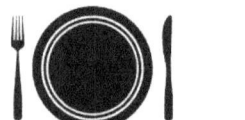

Dates
_____

	BREAKFAST	LUNCH	DINNER	SNACKS
MON				
TUE				
WED				
THU				
FRI				
SAT				
SUN				

FOODS TO AVOID   FOODS TO AVOID   SHOPPING LIST

_____   _____   _____
_____   _____   _____
_____   _____   _____
_____   _____   _____
_____   _____   _____

When dining out, what are some strategies you can use to make kidney stone-friendly choices? List specific dishes or questions you might ask the server.

FOOD TRAKER JOURNAL

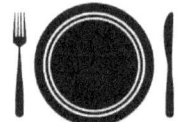

Dates _____

	BREAKFAST	LUNCH	DINNER	SNACKS
MON				
TUE				
WED				
THU				
FRI				
SAT				
SUN				

FOODS TO AVOID   **FOODS TO AVOID**   **SHOPPING LIST**

_____   _____   _____
_____   _____   _____
_____   _____   _____
_____   _____   _____
_____   _____   _____

FOOD TRAKER JOURNAL

Dates _____

	BREAKFAST	LUNCH	DINNER	SNACKS
MON				
TUE				
WED				
THU				
FRI				
SAT				
SUN				

FOODS TO AVOID

_____
_____
_____
_____
_____

FOODS TO AVOID

_____
_____
_____
_____
_____

SHOPPING LIST

_____
_____
_____
_____
_____

SCAN THE QR CODE BELOW TO GET A SURPRISE BONUS!

If you would love to have a one-on-one consultation session with Dr. Kelly Haaland, kindly reach out to us at kellyhaaland2@gmail.com.

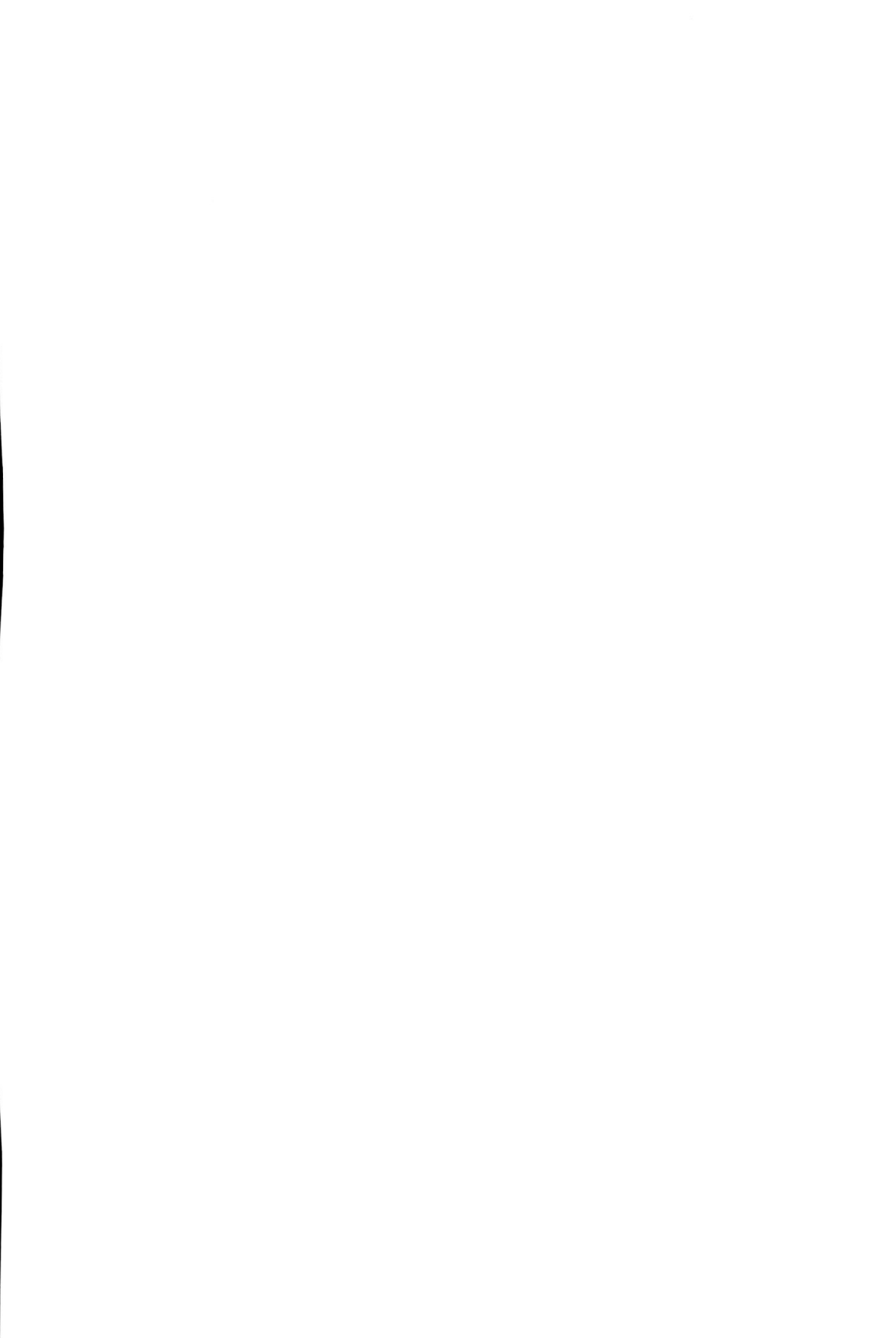

www.ingramcontent.com/pod-product-compliance
Lightning Source LLC
Chambersburg PA
CBHW062107220526
45471CB00010B/3635